Nutrition
CHAMPS

Nutrition
CHAMPS

The Veggie Queen's Guide to
Eating and Cooking for Optimum Health,
Happiness, Energy and Vitality

Jill Nussinow, MS, RD

VEGETARIAN CONNECTION PRESS
SANTA ROSA, CA

2014

Nutrition CHAMPS:

The Veggie Queen's Guide to Eating and Cooking
for Optimum Health, Happiness, Energy and Vitality

Copyright ©2014 Jill Nussinow, MS, RD
All rights reserved.

Published by:
Vegetarian Connection Press
Post Office Box 6042
Santa Rosa, CA 95406-0042
www.vegetarianconnection.com

Cover and Book Design: Patti Buttitta, ButtittaDesign.com
Image Collage, Front Cover: Patti Buttitta
Illustrations: Emily Horstman and Josef Sorenson
Book Production: Phyllis Peterson, MagnoliaStudio.com
Cover Production: Tony Monaco, Media94.com
Photo of Jill Nussinow (back cover): Ed Aiona

ISBN 978-0-9767085-2-0
Library of Congress Control Number: 2014933283
Printed in the United States of America
First Edition

As an eater, please make the wisest
food choices for yourself and the planet.
Our interconnected web of life depends on it.

ACKNOWLEDGMENTS

LIKE ANY BOOK, this book would not have been possible without a host of people to make it a reality. In this case, because this book as a collaboration, I have a lot of people to thank. I want to thank all my friends and colleagues who agreed to contribute their recipes to Nutrition CHAMPS. Their hard work has made this book possible. (For a complete list, please see the "Recipe Contributors" on pages 236-240.)

I have deep gratitude for Dr. Mary Wendt for writing the foreword and for her general kindness and compassion.

A big thank you to my "virtual" intern Sara Turnasella for her research work, backing up the scientific information about each category of food. The studies aren't listed but when you ask a question about a particular food, I will likely be able to put my fingers on related-research due to Sara's for the better part of a year.

I also want to thank my young illustrator, Emily Horstman for her wonderful illustrations. As a side note, if you ever want a killer tattoo, Emily is your woman.

My virtual assistant Nicole Steen has done an amazing job organizing all the recipes and contributors. I honestly do not know how her brain can keep things straight but I am most grateful that she knows her way around an Excel spreadsheet.

A book is just a collection of words without a design team to shape it into book form. I would like to thank Patti Buttitta of Buttitta Design for designing the cover and creating the photographic illustrations, as well as designing the book layout and type treatment. I would like to thank Phyllis Peterson of Magnolia Studio for her keen eye to detail and getting the book into its final production format.

Thank you so much Bonnie Polkinghorn for your proofreader's keen eye. You did more than expected. If any mistakes exist, I take full responsibility. I would also like to thank Tony Monaco for making the critical production adjustments to the cover so that it wraps nicely around the inner pages.

I could not write this book or do any other work without hard working farmers who provide me, and other recipe developers, with the products with which to create. So thank you to every hard working farmer anywhere and everywhere. I give great thanks for the back breaking work that you do. You need to be appreciated and revered. Without farmers, we have no food.

I also always want to be sure to thank my husband who puts up with kitchen messes, constant experimentation, my writing whenever and wherever I am inspired and for allowing me to do the work that I love. Thank you Rick.

ABOUT NUTRITION "CHAMPS"

I derived the acronym "CHAMPS" from the first letter of six plant-based food groups: Cruciferous Vegetables, Herbs, Alliums, Mushrooms, Pulses, Seeds (and Nuts). These plant-based foods cover a lot of nutritional ground. Cruciferous vegetables, which include broccoli, Brussels sprouts, cabbage, cauliflower and turnips (plus others), are known to be cancer protective. Herbs and spices are nutrition powerhouses and make your food taste great. Alliums, onion, garlic, leek, shallot and green onions provide the flavor base for many cooked and raw dishes plus they are packed with phytochemicals for health promotion. Mushrooms are not vegetables, but fungi, which provide valuable fiber and possible cancer-fighting properties. Pulses, which include all types of peas, beans and lentils are protein-packed and contain soluble fiber which might aid in lowering cholesterol. Seeds and nuts add great taste and important fats to round out the plant-based diet. Including the CHAMPS daily will make a difference in your health which will lead to having more happiness, energy and vitality.

— *Jill Nussinow*

TABLE OF CONTENTS

Acknowledgments i

About Nutrition "CHAMPS" ii

Preface v

Foreword by Dr. Mary Clifton, M.D. vii

Introduction ix

Chapter 1: Cruciferous Vegetables 1

Chapter 2: Herbs and Spices 61

Chapter 3: Alliums 93

Chapter 4: Mushrooms 117

Chapter 5: Pulses 147

Chapter 6: Seeds and Nuts 195

End Notes 233

Recipe Contributors 236

Glossary of Terms 241

Ingredient Sources 244

Index 246

Recipes By Author 269

WHILE SOME PEOPLE RECOMMEND that you eat certain foods each day such as Joel Fuhrman, M.D.'s G-BOMBS, I think that it is more important to make sure that you get a wide variety of highly nutritious, and tasty, foods. There are many more foods than those that I will be discussing and focusing on in this book that have great nutrition value. I wanted this book to be accessible and not be bogged down with cited studies (there are more than 5600 peer reviewed studies for turmeric alone), so I chose not to include every food that could positively impact your nutrition life and health.

If you include most of the Nutrition CHAMPS foods daily, you ought to be fine, as long as the other foods that join the bunch are more nutritious than not. If you choose to eat less nutritious foods, that is your choice.

The one thing that I have always loved about eating (at least here in the U.S.) is that we have many choices for what to put in our mouths. This is one area of your life where you get to make the decisions.

This is NOT a rule book although I have some eating rules which you can read below. Since so many people contributed to the making of this book, I didn't do a lot of recipe editing. I took the recipes that were offered. Some might use more oil than what I would usually use (which in many cases is none), more sugar or more salt. Feel free to adjust the recipes to your specific way of eating. While making recipes that contain the "best" ingredients makes sense, it also makes great sense to me that food ought to taste great. While this type of food "is good medicine," I don't want it to taste that way.

The focus is on the CHAMPS foods and not other foods which might also be nutrition powerhouses such as sea vegetables, land vegetables other than the ones discussed herein, whole grains, berries and other fruit. While there are superfoods, many foods are super without that moniker. My motto, "If it comes from a plant, there is likely good nutrition in it." Some foods, though, have better nutrition than others. I say, "Eat a huge variety of foods but make the CHAMPS ingredients your foundation."

Here is my short list of rules:

Don't eat what you don't like but be sure that you truly don't like it. If you had asked me years ago if I liked mustard, I would have definitely said NO. That has changed. So, give food a chance. Try preparing, or cooking it, in more than one way to see if you like a particular food.

Don't use what you don't have. Read through the recipes before you attempt to cook them. If you end up without an ingredient and it's not the most important ingredient in the recipe, the recipe will likely turn out just fine. Or find a good substitute for what you are missing. I have made my Rich Tahini Gravy without tahini and it was still good. Funny, huh?

When you eat something cooked, eat something raw. I am by no means a raw foodist. But my gut instinct tells me that we need to eat raw food when we eat cooked food. That can be as small as chopped herbs on top of your dish or it might be some fermented vegetables to accompany your cooked dish to bolster the flavor and texture. Or maybe you'd rather go the big green salad route which is another one of my favorite raw foods. The choices are up to you.

Eating Tips for Optimum Health

Below are helpful reminders for planning your meals:

A large green leafy salad daily is an important addition to your diet. A good rule is pair a cooked dish with something raw, even as a garnish.

More brightly colored vegetables contain more phytochemicals.

The vegetables in season provide the lowest cost, best taste and most nutrition. If possible grow your own or shop at a farmers' market or store with high produce turnover.

Fruit is also a great source of fiber. Be careful not to overeat in-season fruit and dried fruit. If someone has cancer, avoiding all sugars might be the smartest move.

Add healthier fats such as olives and avocados in moderation.

If you eat grains, choose whole grains instead of whole grain bread. In general, the less processed the food, the better.

Eating well for health does not have to be difficult, expensive or boring. Food should and can taste great!

— *Jill Nussinow*

FOREWORD

JILL IS RIGHT. The best messages are clear, easy to remember, and easy to understand. That's why I think Jill has hit a home run with her newest book, *Nutrition CHAMPS*. Eating healthy is easy and delicious, when you're cooking recipes collected from her variety of great contributors. These recipes can prevent you from suffering with disease and reverse illnesses you already battle. After a very scary doctor visit seven years ago, I personally cured my high blood sugar and elevated cholesterol with recipes just like the ones in this book, changing my body a meal at a time. I wish I would have had this handy guide available to me when I was fighting for my health so many years ago.

Jill is an expert. She's especially knowledgeable in the field of mushrooms and their nutritional and medicinal qualities. Mushrooms are immune boosting, cancer fighting, and a great source of Vitamin D, all while being low in calories. She's been foraging and cooking and speaking about these powerful health promoters for fifteen years. Consuming mushrooms regularly is associated with decreased risk of breast, stomach, and colorectal cancers. In one recent Chinese study, women who ate about one mushroom per day had a 64% decreased risk of breast cancer. Even more dramatic protection was gained by women who ate 10 grams of mushrooms and drank green tea daily — an 89% decrease in risk for premenopausal women, and 82% for postmenopausal women. Mushrooms contain aromatase inhibitors, compounds that block the production of estrogen and are the active ingredients in cancer prevention pharmaceutical agents like Tamoxifen. Different mushrooms have different nutritional and health promoting properties, so consuming a wide variety is an even better idea than consuming just one type. However, even the humble white button mushroom you can purchase from the largest chain grocery boosts immunity against common colds and flu for up to two weeks after ingestion.

However, in the act of tearing something apart, you may lose its meaning. Foods are not simply component parts of lesser or greater nutritional value. The only proven way to benefit from the nutrients in foods is to eat the whole foods. While food science is interesting, it is not valuable to rely on individual nutrients in supplements to protect your valuable body. All the doctors and scientists on this great planet can theorize about why whole foods are valuable for you, but the best advice is to eat the whole food. CHAMPS is an acronym you can use to remember the most nutrient-dense, health-promoting foods on the planet. These are the foods you should eat every single day, and they should make up a significant proportion of your diet *(See: http://www.drfuhrman.com/library/foodpyramid.aspx)*. These foods are extremely effective at preventing chronic disease and promoting health and longevity.

Adding the foods recommended in this book regularly to your diet will promote your best health and slim your waistline. When I first met Jill at a conference last year, I was impressed by her passion, and also by the radiant health that shines all around her. After you meet her, you'll want to follow her diet and lifestyle too, just to get those great vibes going in your own life. This book will work for you. Jill will help you reshape your body. You can be the healthiest you've ever been by following the advice and recipes contained in Nutrition CHAMPS.

My very best wishes to you! May you reach all your health and wellness goals!

—Dr. Mary (Clifton) Wendt, M.D.

References:

Hong SA, Kim K, Nam SJ, et al. A case-control study on the dietary intake of mushrooms and breast cancer risk among Korean women. Int J Cancer 2008;122:919-923.

Shin A, Kim J, Lim SY, et al. Dietary mushroom intake and the risk of breast cancer based on hormone receptor status. Nutr Cancer 2010;62:476-483.

Zhang M, Huang J, Xie X, et al. Dietary intakes of mushrooms and green tea combine to reduce the risk of breast cancer in Chinese women. Int J Cancer 2009;124:1404-1408.

Hara M, Hanaoka T, Kobayashi M, et al. Cruciferous vegetables, mushrooms, and gastrointestinal cancer risks in a multicenter, hospital-based case-control study in Japan. Nutr Cancer 2003;46:138-147.

Chen S, Oh SR, Phung S, et al. Anti-aromatase activity of phytochemicals in white button mushrooms (Agaricus bisporus). Cancer Res 2006;66: 12026-12034.

Jeong SC, Koyyalamudi SR, Pang G, Dietary Intake of Agaricus Bisporus White Button Mushrooms Accelerates Salivary Immunoglobulin A Secretion in Healthy Volunteers, Nutrition 2012, Ma;28(5):527-31.

INTRODUCTION

I HAVE BEEN A REGISTERED DIETITIAN for more than 30 years. During this time, I have done individual counseling... but most of all, I have taught people how to eat and cook — in a way similar to how I eat.

The idea for this book was sparked by a talk that Dr. Joel Fuhrman did in Santa Rosa, California in February 2012. He spoke about his *Super Immunity* book. Most of what he spoke about is what I have been preaching and teaching for my entire career, especially the last ten years. When Dr. Fuhrman mentioned G-BOMBS (which he has now changed to GBOMBS) I had to write that down. Then I had to study that acronym for more than a week to remember what those letters stood for (greens, onions, mushrooms, beans, berries, seeds).

While I agree with the message behind GOMBBS, I cannot promote that word and the reason is because it's not a word, certainly not one that I have ever heard in my years on earth. Perhaps, it's a doctor word. I honestly don't know.

The more that I thought about the acronym, the more it didn't make sense to me. So I came up with my own acronym CHAMPS which echoes Dr. Fuhrman's in some ways and deviates (or departs) in others.

I want people to remember what the letters spell because I believe that including these foods as part of your regular eating will give you more energy and keep you feeling great, helping you maintain your health.

Even though we are all different, eating this way has worked for me and I am pretty sure that it will work for you. My predilection for vegetables, and fruit, existed even when I was a child. I can recall being a 4-year-old and shelling peas in the summer time. I am sure that many never made it to the bowl that my mom gave me. I also have always loved eating red peppers. My mom planted them but they were hot and made me sick but that still didn't deter me. I had a crying fit when we moved from our house when I was five because I had to leave my beloved "fruit cocktail tree." I have since recovered from that incident and gone on to eat even more vegetables.

My grandfather was one of the first people to follow the Kempner Rice Diet after he had a heart attack in his mid-40s. My grandmother cooked "special" food for him. Whenever they came over to eat I would want to eat my "Poppa's" food because it tasted so good. He always had baked potatoes and tomatoes, and other fresh vegetables.

I had my food likes and dislikes and one food that I came to despise was meat. I guess that it was a good thing that I liked so many other foods. I was a teenager when I stopped eating meat. I easily gave up eating it. No matter what your age, cutting meat out of your diet is a good idea. For many people the issue becomes which foods stand in for the meat. This book will give you a good idea of those foods so that you can make good choices.

I recently met a man who was doing 21-day juice fasts and feeling great. As soon as he was done he would go back to his "regular eating" and once again he would feel awful. He said that he did this for 3 years until he had his "Aha" moment. He had recorded a PBS show for his brother featuring Neal Barnard, M.D., speaking about diabetes. When his brother still hadn't watched the recording a month later, he watched it. This is when he heard that you could cut out the meat and be okay. He found the answer to his eating dilemma. Now he follows a plant-based diet and feels great all the time.

I want to encourage you to eat as many plant foods as possible. Not all of them are included in this book but reading this and incorporating my recommendations and recipes from amazing recipe developers will get you off to a more-than-good start to becoming a nutrition champ. I would love to see millions of people becoming nutrition CHAMPS which will lead to improved health and feeling great. Without your health, it's hard to enjoy life.

— *Jill Nussinow*

*Here's to great eating
and cooking.*

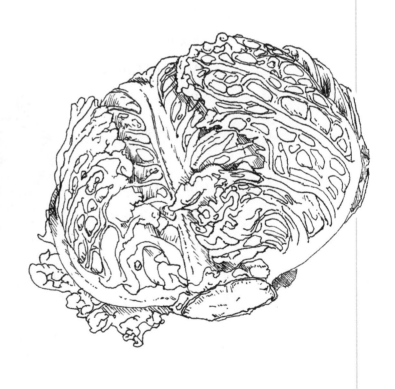

CHAMPS

Cruciferous Vegetables Included

Arugula

Bok Choy

Broccoli

Broccoli Rabe

Brussels Sprouts

Cabbage

Cauliflower

Collard Greens

Horseradish

Kale

Kohlrabi

Mustard Greens

Radish

Rutabaga

Tatsoi

Turnips

Turnip Greens

Watercress

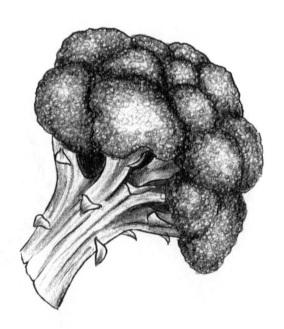

CHAPTER 1

Cruciferous Vegetables

KALE SEEMS AS IF it may be the "new black." I am here to open the curtain and expose the rainbow of choices that are almost as good as kale and can keep you eating a new vegetable daily for a couple of weeks. While we think of green vegetables as offering the most health, recent research reveals that white vegetables such as cauliflower, turnips, kohlrabi and daikon radish, all crucifers, and garlic and onion, two allium family vegetables, have plenty to offer nutritionally. Cruciferous vegetables contain an exclusive compound of phytonutrients: the glucosinolates. These likely help with cancer protection and prevention. The glucosinonales produce myrosinase which is beneficial. Some of the myrosinase will convert to isothiocyanates. (You do not have to remember any of this science.)

These vegetables are low in calories and nutrient rich with vitamins C, K, A as beta-carotene and folic acid as folate, as well as antioxidants which allow them to keep inflammation at bay, while detoxifying our bodies. (The science is long and deep and I won't go into it here.)

The best way to eat these vegetables is to eat them raw, ferment them or cook them quickly by pressure cooking or steaming for less than 10 minutes. There is some evidence that longer cooking denatures the beneficial compounds. There is also evidence that chopping the vegetables helps you get more of the beneficial compounds although they ought to be cooked or eaten immediately rather than letting them sit around which might yield fewer beneficial compounds. If the fiber from these plants makes it intact to your large intestine, they are good for making beneficial bacteria and other compounds which are health promoting.

Crucifers are members of the Brassica family of vegetables. Crucifer means cross and they either grow in a cross pattern or their flowers look like crosses. I think that they are truly amazing because there are so many of them. They include leaves, buds and roots. Some of the vegetables provide double duty, giving you more to eat such as turnips or radishes, which also have edible greens. The list to the left is comprehensive but, of course, does not include every vegetable. For instance, some eaten in other parts of the world are not on this list.

Arugula and Herb Pesto

—JILL NUSSINOW—

This is a creamy pesto dip for raw vegetables. We will use what is fresh from the garden. If you want to use oil, omit the white beans or tofu but the calories will get much higher.

Serves 4

3 cloves minced garlic

3 cups chopped arugula

1 cup chopped flat leaf parsley

2–3 tablespoons pine nuts

½ cup cooked white beans or silken tofu

1–2 tablespoons light miso (to taste)

¼ to ⅓ cup water or broth

2 tablespoons nutritional yeast

2 tablespoons olive oil, optional if not using beans or tofu

In food processor, combine everything except water or broth. Pulse till finely minced. With machine running, slowly add water until reaches desired consistency.

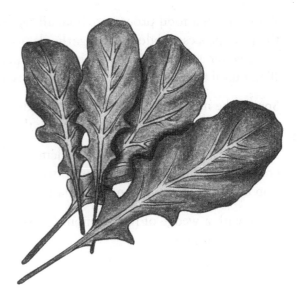

Lemon-Pepper Arugula Pizza
with White Bean Basil Sauce

—JAIME KARPOVICH—

This simple "cheese" and arugula combine to make pizzas with pizazz.

Serves 6

6 whole grain pitas (or cooked pizza dough)

1½ cups cooked cannellini beans (one can if using canned)

1 bunch basil leaves

3 cloves garlic

Juice of ½ lemon

½ cup nutritional yeast

Salt, to taste

2–3 cups fresh arugula

Juice of 1 lemon, plus fresh lemon wedges for garnish

Fresh cracked black pepper

Put beans in a food processor. Take all the leaves of a bunch of basil and add to the food processor, along with garlic, lemon juice, nutritional yeast and salt. (Add water 1 tablespoon at a time if you need to help blend ingredients.) Blend until smooth, stopping to scrape down the sides if needed.

Spread the mixture on top of the pita or dough, making a thick layer of "cheese." (If you have more "cheese" than you need, the rest can go in the fridge for a few days.)

Put arugula in a mixing bowl with lemon juice and mix to coat. Add some fresh cracked pepper (and salt if desired) to make the arugula as peppery as you like. Top the pizzas with lemony arugula mixture.

Serve with a wedge of fresh lemon. Guests can use wedges to add fresh lemon juice to their own pizzas.

Shangri-La Soup

—VICTORIA MORAN—

Among the ageless women and men I know, a percentage too high to be happenstance attribute their youthfulness to a high-raw, plant-based diet, so I'd like to share with you here a raw soup — gazpacho isn't the only one! Raw soups are creamy and tangy and when I have one for lunch, I feel as if I couldn't be taking better care of myself — because that's the truth. This recipe, named for the legendary land of eternal youth, makes two appetizer-sized servings, or lunch for one healthy, hungry person.

Serves 1–2

8 baby carrots

6 cherry tomatoes, or 1 medium tomato

4 scant cups organic arugula

¾ teaspoon Italian herbs (sometimes called "Italian seasoning")

½ teaspoon onion powder

⅛ teaspoon lemon pepper

⅛ teaspoon cayenne

1–2 tablespoons lemon juice

½ medium avocado, chopped or mashed

Chopped red bell pepper to garnish, optional

Chop carrots and tomatoes in food processor. Add half the arugula and a little water to process until it's a soupy slurry.

Add remaining arugula, spices, and lemon juice (start with 1 tablespoon; if you like a tart flavor as I do, you'll want to add more), plus more water to process to a chunky consistency. Then add the avocado and process briefly.

Garnish with chopped red pepper if you like.

Summer Arugula Salad
with Lemon Tahini Dressing

—CHRISTY MORGAN—

The bitterness of arugula is tempered with this tasty dressing and the sweetness of strawberries and sweet red pepper.

Serves 4

SALAD

4–5 cups arugula, packed

1 (14-ounce) can chickpeas, rinsed and drained

7 strawberries, washed, topped and sliced

1 small red bell pepper, thinly sliced

DRESSING

1 teaspoon lemon zest

¼ cup lemon juice

¼ cup water, or more as needed

3 tablespoons tahini, roasted preferred

1 tablespoon nutritional yeast

1 tablespoon maple syrup, or more to taste

1 tablespoon red wine vinegar

1 teaspoon garlic powder

Sea salt and black pepper, to taste

Cayenne, to taste

Toss all salad ingredients into a large bowl.

Mix all dressing ingredients in a blender or whisk by hand in a small bowl until smooth. Add more water as needed. Season with sea salt to taste.

Drizzle dressing over salad if serving immediately. Or, put into an airtight container and refrigerate for later use.

Bok Choy Ginger Dizzle

—SHARON GREENSPAN—

Bok choy is a powerhouse of Vitamin C, calcium and beta-carotene. But I love it because it has a variety of textures. The stalks are crunchy and sweet. The leaves are deep green and tender. It's like getting two veggies in one!

Serves 4–6

- ½ cup zucchini
- 2 teaspoons crushed hot pepper
- 2 teaspoons grated ginger
- 1½ tablespoons chopped red onion
- 2 tablespoons lemon juice
- Dash of salt (sea, Celtic or Himalayan)
- ¼ cup water or to desired consistency
- ½ head of medium-sized bok choy, chopped to equal 3–4 cups
- 1–2 cucumbers, peeled

Blend all ingredients except bok choy and cucumber until smooth. Pour over bok choy and mix well. Add cucumbers and lightly stir. Allow to marinate at least 20 minutes.

Sesame Bok Choy Shiitake Stir Fry

—JENN LYNSKEY—

This dish comes together quickly and works with either noodles or rice depending on your mood.

Serves 2

- 2–3 small bok choy sliced into bite-sized pieces
- 1 cup shiitake mushrooms, sliced
- 1 tablespoon miso paste
- 1 tablespoon tahini
- 1 tablespoon soy sauce or tamari
- 1 tablespoon sake or mirin
- 1 tablespoon rice vinegar
- Black and white sesame seeds for garnish

Blend together miso, tahini, soy sauce, sake or mirin, and rice vinegar.

In a sauté pan, add the bok choy, mushrooms, and sauce and cook until heated and the mushrooms are soft and bok choy is a little wilted.

Serve over noodles or rice and top with black and white sesame seeds.

Bok Choy, Green Garlic and Greens
with Sweet Ginger Sauce

—JILL NUSSINOW—

This tastes great and can be served with soba noodles or colored rice, or your favorite grain or noodle. This dish is a more than a bit beyond the ordinary.

Serves 4

1 tablespoon oil

½ leek, sliced

2 medium garlic cloves, crushed with flat side of a knife

1 1-inch thick slice of ginger root, halved and smashed with flat side of a chef's knife blade

1 teaspoon minced ginger

2 tablespoons tamari or soy sauce

1 teaspoon sesame oil

Salt and ground black pepper

1½ pounds mustard or other greens (1 large bunch), washed well, leaves trimmed from ribs and cut into 2-inch pieces

3–4 stems green garlic, sliced into 2-inch diagonal pieces

1–2 cups sliced bok choy

1–2 cups pea shoots

3 tablespoons toasted sesame seeds

Heat the oil in a sauté pan over medium high heat. Add the leeks, garlic and ginger.

Sauté for 1–2 minutes. Add the mustard and other greens.

Add the broth and simmer for 2–3 minutes. Add the remaining ingredients except for sesame seeds.

Cook until greens are cooked through and the liquid is almost absorbed.

Sprinkle with the sesame seeds.

Yam Boats
with Chickpeas, Bok Choy and Cashew Dill Sauce
—CHRISTY MORGAN—

Yams come in over 200 varieties! Not only are they a good source of Vitamin C they are high in Vitamin B6 and potassium. And they are naturally sweet! So if you are trying to get off sugar it's a good idea to increase the sweet vegetables in your diet. Feel free to up or change the spices and if you want to make the filling spicy throw in some cayenne! This is great served with a side of quinoa.

Serves 4

2 large jewel yams

½ cup vegetable broth or water

2 tablespoons chopped shallot

1 tablespoon fresh ginger

2 teaspoons garlic powder

1 teaspoon coriander

Pinch sea salt

2 cups packed chopped bok choy

2 cups cooked chickpeas

Sea salt and black pepper, to taste

CASHEW DILL SAUCE

1 cup raw cashews, soaked 1 hour

½ cup unsweetened non-dairy milk + 2 tablespoons

¼ cup chopped fresh dill

2 tablespoons nutritional yeast

1 tablespoon lemon juice

1 tablespoon apple cider vinegar

2 teaspoons garlic powder

Sea salt, if needed

Preheat oven to 400°F. Cut yams in half and place on a lined cookie sheet face down. Bake for about 25 minutes until fork tender. Meanwhile, make your filling and the Cashew Dill Sauce.

For the filling: In a skillet heat the vegetable broth until bubbly. Add the shallots, ginger, salt and spices and sauté for a few minutes. Add bok choy and chickpeas. then cover with a lid. Cook for a few minutes, stirring occasionally. Scrape out most the innards of the yams and stir into the mixture. Season with sea salt and pepper to taste.

For the sauce: Blend ingredients in a blender or food processor until well combined. Season to taste.

To serve: Fill the yam boats with the vegetable filling, then drizzle with Cashew Dill Sauce. Serve immediately with a side of brown rice or quinoa.

Baked Broccoli Burgers

—NIKKI HANEY—

These Baked Broccoli Burgers provide an easy and delicious way to add fiber, vitamins and minerals to your diet. They're packed with vitamins A, B, C and K, as well as fiber, iron, calcium, magnesium and beta-carotene. These burgers work well with a variety of toppings including tahini sauce, hummus and ketchup. The broccoli mixture can be stored in an airtight container and refrigerated for 2–3 days before shaping and baking.

Serves 4

⅓ cup dry couscous

1 cup water

1½ cups broccoli florets

2 teaspoons olive oil

½ cup chopped scallions

½ cup chopped yellow onion

2 teaspoons ground cumin

1 (15-ounce) can of chickpeas, rinsed and drained

1 tablespoon sesame tahini

½ cup panko bread crumbs

Preheat your oven to 400°F. If you can, do the first three steps at the same time in order to speed up the prep time.

In a small pot, bring the water and couscous to a boil. Remove from heat immediately and allow the couscous to sit in the pot for 10 minutes, soaking up the water.

Steam the broccoli in a steamer for 5–7 minutes (or use a microwave) you just want the broccoli to be soft in the end).

In a skillet, heat the olive oil over medium heat and add in the onion and scallions, stirring occasionally for 3–5 minutes until the onion softens. Remove from heat and stir in the cumin.

Gather your couscous, broccoli, onion mix, chickpeas and sesame tahini and combine together in a food processor. Pour the mixture into a bowl and stir in the bread crumbs. Form it into patties and place the patties on a cookie sheet lined with foil.

Bake for 50 minutes, turning the patties over halfway through. You'll know they are done when the tops begin to brown.

Top your burgers with your favorite sauce, a couple of pickles, tomato and lettuce.

Creamy Dreamy Broccoli Soup

—JILL NUSSINOW—

There are a number of ways to make creamed soups without the cream or dairy. In this case, we'll use cooked potato blended with boxed silken tofu and soy milk to add a creamy mouth feel. If you don't want to use soy, then add 3 tablespoons of powdered cashews which also makes the soup creamy. You can do this same cream technique with almost any vegetable that you want to turn into soup. Add herbs in season such as thyme, lemon thyme, tarragon or your favorite for even more flavor.

Serves 4

1 head broccoli, or as much as you want

1 medium onion, chopped

½ (12.3 ounce) box *Mori-Nu* firm silken tofu

½ cup soy or other non-dairy milk

2 medium potatoes

3 cups vegetable broth or water

1 tablespoon parsley or chives and their flowers, for garnish

Salt and pepper, to taste

Remove stems from broccoli and peel. Cut into small pieces. Cut the rest of the head into florets, reserving a few for garnish.

Heat a saucepan over medium heat. Add the onion and sauté for about 3 minutes. Cut potatoes into eights. Add to the onion along with the broccoli stems and vegetable broth. Cook about 10 minutes until the potatoes start getting soft. If the potatoes are not softened, cook another 5 minutes. Remove 1 cup of this mixture and set aside. Then add the broccoli florets to the pot. Cook for 5 minutes until the florets are cooked through.

Purée the tofu and soy milk in the food processor until perfectly creamy.

Using a hand blender, if you have one, purée the soup mixture in the pot until almost smooth. (If you don't have a hand blender, use a blender (very carefully) or a food processor to blend.) Stir in the tofu purée.

Heat gently, but do not allow to boil or the tofu mixture will curdle. Season with salt and pepper. Garnish with parsley or chives and their flowers and the remaining broccoli florets.

Fennel with Broccoli, Zucchini and Peppers

—MARY MCDOUGALL—

Many of you may be unfamiliar with using fennel, but this dish has so much flavor you will wonder why you have never tried this vegetable before. Most supermarkets carry fennel bulbs in the fresh produce section and many farmers' markets also have it.

Serves 4

2 cups sliced fresh fennel
(see the *Hints* below)

1 cup broccoli florets

1 cup sliced zucchini

½ cup coarsely chopped red bell pepper

2 cups vegetable broth

Freshly ground black pepper

Place the vegetables and 1 cup of the broth in a large non-stick sauté pan. Grind some fresh black pepper over the vegetables. Cover and steam for 5 minutes, then remove the cover and continue to cook, stirring frequently until most of the broth is absorbed and the vegetables are beginning to stick to the bottom of the pan.

Add another ½ cup of the broth and a few more twists of pepper. Continue to cook and stir, uncovered, until broth is again absorbed and vegetables begin to stick again.

Add the remaining broth and more black pepper. Continue to cook until broth is absorbed again. Taste and add more black pepper if desired before serving.

Hints:

Fresh fennel is sometimes sold under the name anise, with several inches of fine leafy fronds attached. Cut the fronds off at the top of the bulb, trim the root end, cut the entire bulb in half lengthwise and then slice thinly. Two medium-sized bulbs should yield about 2 cups sliced. If you have a bit more than 2 cups, just use the extra amount in this recipe.

Slice the zucchini in half lengthwise and then slice thinly. One zucchini should yield about 1 cup.

One half of a red bell pepper should yield about ½ cup of ½-inch size pieces.

Romanesco Broccoli Sauce

—JILL NUSSINOW—

I used to serve this sauce over pasta but these days I like it better served over brown rice or quinoa. Romanesco broccoli is really a cauliflower. Don't ask me to explain its name. Even with the confusion, I think that it's a wonderful vegetable — beautiful to look at and very tasty.

Serves 4

1 tablespoon oil, optional

½ medium onion, diced to equal 1 cup

2–3 cloves garlic, minced

4 cups Romanesco broccoli florets

6–8 sundried tomatoes, rehydrated in hot water and cut into slivers

1 teaspoon crushed red pepper flakes

½ cup vegetable broth

2 tablespoons capers

1 tablespoon Meyer, or other, lemon juice

2 tablespoons chopped Italian parsley

Freshly ground black pepper

Heat the oil, if using, in a medium skillet. Add the onion and sauté over medium heat for 3 minutes, adding broth if onion starts to stick.

After 3 minutes, add the garlic and broccoli florets and sauté for another 3 minutes, adding broth, as necessary.

Add the remaining ingredients except the lemon juice and parsley. Cook until the broccoli is tender.

Add the lemon juice and top with parsley. Add pepper, to taste.

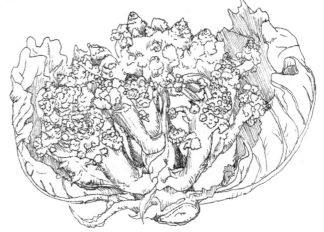

Stir-Fry Toppings

—ELLEN JONES—

When we hear the advice, "Eat the colors of the rainbow," we often assume this mainly applies to vibrant colors of fresh, raw fruits and vegetables. But it is important to keep gorgeous colors in cooked food too, which is your insurance policy to resist disease with a recipe packed with anti-oxidants. The key to keeping color in cooked food is not overcooking. If you can use a food processor, you'll have this done in no time. But even if you don't, this should take no more than 20 minutes max to prepare, and another 10 minutes to cook.

Serves 6-8

½ cup dry lentils

1¼ cup liquid vegetable broth

½ head broccoli, cut into florets

4 medium turnips and greens, cut into small chunks and thin strips

1 large portabello mushroom, cut into small chunks

1 medium carrot, cut into thin rounds

¼ head red cabbage, sliced into thin shreds (approximately 1–2 cups)

1 orange or yellow pepper, cored, seeded and diced

1 medium summer squash, cut into thin rounds

1 medium zucchini, cut into thin rounds

10–12 small cherry or Roma tomatoes, cut in halves

2 tablespoons fresh oregano, chopped

2 tablespoons fresh parsley, chopped

1 tablespoon sesame seeds

2 tablespoons onion flakes

2 tablespoons garlic chips or 1 tablespoon garlic powder

1 cup cooked brown rice or your favorite whole grain

In a small pot, add the lentils and 1 cup of the liquid vegetable broth. Bring to a boil. Reduce heat, cover and simmer for 20–30 minutes until the lentils are cooked.

While the lentils are cooking, in a large pot or wok, add the remaining broth along with the broccoli, turnips, mushrooms, carrot and cabbage. Cook over low heat, stirring to keep vegetables from sticking, until they are just starting to become soft. Add the turnip greens, yellow pepper, squash, zucchini and tomatoes. Cook for another 5–10 minutes until all the vegetables are soft, but not mushy. Sprinkle the sesame seeds, onion flakes and garlic chips over the mixture during the last minute of cooking to add extra protein and crunch. Stir well. Serve over the rice.

Thai-Inspired Broccoli Slaw

—JILL NUSSINOW—

There is nothing wrong with plain broccoli but this recipe elevates broccoli to new heights. If you want this to be a main meal salad, add some baked tofu or seitan cubes. Don't let the long ingredient list stop you from making this. This tastes great right away but sometimes tastes even better the next day, if you have any leftover.

Freeze the leftover coconut milk in ice cube or other small amounts so that you won't have to open a new can every time you need coconut milk. It will last about 3 months in the freezer.

Serves 4

- 1 large bunch broccoli, about 2 pounds
- 1 tablespoon finely chopped fresh lemongrass
- 1 kaffir lime leaf, if available or 1 teaspoon lime zest and ½ teaspoon juice
- ¼ cup boiling water or stock
- ¼ cup peanut butter
- 1 tablespoon rice vinegar
- 1 teaspoon grated ginger
- 1 clove garlic, crushed
- ¼ teaspoon crushed red pepper flakes
- ¼ cup lite or regular coconut milk
- 1 tablespoon *Bragg Liquid Aminos* or tamari
- 1–2 tablespoons lime juice
- Sweetener to taste
- 2 tablespoons finely chopped roasted red pepper
- ¼ cup minced fresh cilantro
- 2 tablespoons finely chopped green onions

Cut the broccoli into small florets. Peel the stalks and cut them into slices ½-inch thick. Steam over boiling water for 3–5 minutes until tender. Remove from heat and put into a bowl. Refrigerate to cool until ready to use.

Pour the boiling water over the lemongrass and kaffir lime leaf in a heatproof bowl. Let sit for at least 10 minutes to extract flavor. Strain the lemongrass water and put the liquid into a blender. Combine with the remaining ingredients except the cilantro and green onions. Blend until smooth. Taste and adjust the seasonings.

Pour dressing over the broccoli. Add the roasted red pepper and toss. Garnish with the cilantro and green onions.

Zesty Broccoli Rabe
with Chickpeas and Pasta

—BEVERLY BENNETT—

The bitter flavor of broccoli rabe is further accentuated by cooking it in vegetable broth with chickpeas, onion, and a generous amount of garlic and crushed red pepper flakes in this hearty pasta dish.

Serves 6

8 ounces whole-grain pasta (such as fusilli, penne, rigatoni, or ziti)

1 cup low-sodium vegetable broth

½ cup diced red or yellow onion

1 medium bunch broccoli rabe (about 1½ pound), coarsely cut into approximately 1-inch pieces

2 tablespoons minced garlic

1 teaspoon dried oregano

1 teaspoon crushed red pepper flakes

1 (15-ounce) can chickpeas, drained and rinsed, or 1½ cups

⅓ cup chopped fresh basil or parsley

1½ tablespoons nutritional yeast flakes, plus additional for garnishing

Sea salt

Freshly ground black pepper

Fill a large saucepan two-thirds full of water, and bring to a boil over medium-high heat. Add pasta and cook, stirring occasionally, according to the package directions or until al dente. Remove from the heat. Drain the pasta in a colander, but do not rinse.

Meanwhile, place a large nonstick skillet over medium heat. Add ½ cup vegetable broth and onion, cook, stirring occasionally, for 3 minutes. Add the remaining ½ cup vegetable broth, broccoli rabe, garlic, oregano, and red pepper flakes and cook, stirring occasionally, for 3–5 minutes or until broccoli rabe is crisp-tender.

Add the chickpeas, cooked pasta, chopped basil, and nutritional yeast flakes and stir well to combine. Season with salt and pepper to taste. Remove from the heat.

Serve hot and top individual servings with additional nutritional yeast flakes as desired.

Cream of Brussels Sprouts Soup
with Vegan Cream Sauce

—CARRIE FORREST—

This recipe makes a lot of soup, so get out your largest pot. You'll be happy you made it, though, because it is delicious and nutritious and the leftovers freeze beautifully. The flavor is sweet from the butternut squash, but it is incredibly healthy (and green!) due to the sprouts and spinach.

Serves 10–12

SOUP

1 pound button mushrooms
(about 2 cups, chopped)
1 large onion, chopped
1 large tomato, chopped
2 pounds butternut squash, chopped
1 tablespoon dried marjoram
1 tablespoon no-salt seasoning
1 teaspoon turmeric

6 cups no-sodium or reduced-sodium vegetable broth
2 pounds Brussels sprouts, sliced
1 pound fresh baby spinach
Fresh lemon juice (optional)

VEGAN CREAM SAUCE

1 cup raw cashews
1 cup unsweetened soy milk

Place an extra-large pot on the stove and turn on medium heat for a few minutes. Once the bottom of the pot is hot, add onions and reduce heat to medium-low. Stir onions frequently until they start to cook, about 2–3 minutes. Add mushrooms and continue to stir frequently. Don't allow the onions to burn.

Add chopped tomato for additional moisture and cook for an additional 2 minutes. Add spices and butternut squash to pot, topped with vegetable broth. Bring to a boil on high heat and then turn back heat to simmer for 5 minutes.

Pour in sliced Brussels sprouts and add additional water or broth as needed to cover. Put lid on pot (slightly ajar) and simmer for 10 minutes or until squash and sprouts are cooked through. Add spinach a minute or two before the end of cooking.

Using a high-speed blender, batch process the soup until it is blended, being very careful not to burn yourself. Stir in Vegan Cream Sauce (see instructions below) and serve hot with a squeeze of fresh lemon juice for added flavor. Freeze or refrigerate leftovers.

For Vegan Cream Sauce: Combine ingredients in a high-speed blender and process until smooth. Sauce will thicken as it sits.

Brussels Sprouts —
The Vegetable We Love to Say We Hate

Shortly before moving to Sonoma County in the late 1980s, I was invited as part of a select group of dietitians, just one from each state, to attend a conference in Minnesota. It was designed to help us learn how to disseminate nutrition information to our local community. I decided that I wanted to promote vegetables. (You can see that I have been at this for a long time.)

I developed a brochure about Brussels sprouts as a mock-up of my idea. I now realize that I was out of my mind to try promoting a vegetable that most people think that they hate. The reality is far different. In fact, the last time that I prepared Brussels sprouts at one of my cooking classes they were gobbled up quickly. When I was pitching the idea of eating Brussels sprouts, some members of The Sonoma County Farmlands Group affectionately referred to me as the "Brussels sprouts woman." That was fine with me. Since then I have come to realize that dislike for this vegetable arises out of improper preparation and cooking procedures. Undercooked sprouts do not taste good. But when cooked to perfection, and there are a number of ways to do this, they are delectable.

No matter how you cook the sprouts, start by cutting off any old outer leaves and the bottom of the stem. Make an X in the stem end. Since this is a cruciferous vegetable, which means it grows like a cross, X marks the spot. Steam the sprouts in the microwave or a pot for just a couple of minutes or more, depending on the rest of the cooking treatment.

One of my favorite ways to cook Brussels sprouts is by cutting them in half and sautéing them in either a dry pan or with a touch of oil, with something sweet like orange juice or maple syrup, and tossing in some chopped nuts. They are also amazing pressure cooked in vegetable broth for just a couple of minutes. Or you can halve them, mix with a little olive oil and put them on a baking sheet. Bake at 400°F for about 20 minutes until cooked through. Season any way you like.

If I am going to cut away the stem and use only the leaves, then I do not precook but add liquid in the cooking process to help assure that the leaves are cooked thoroughly. Brussels sprouts are wonderful paired with nuts, such as almonds, chestnuts and hazelnuts (also known as filberts), which arrive on the scene around the same time, from late fall into the winter.

Be creative and make up your own recipe for one of America's most hated vegetables. You just might have to cross it off your "do not like" list.

— Jill Nussinow

Roasted Turmeric Brussels Sprouts
with Hemp Seeds on Arugula

—AMIE VALPONE—

This recipe is a great-tasting CHAMPS powerhouse. Roasting often brings out the sweetness of the sprouts.

Serves 2

1 pound large Brussels sprouts, halved

2 tablespoons extra virgin olive oil

¼ teaspoon sea salt

¼ teaspoon freshly ground pepper

¼ teaspoon turmeric

2 teaspoons hemp seeds

2 teaspoons balsamic vinegar

Preheat oven to 350°F. In a large bowl, toss Brussels sprouts with oil and hemp seeds, turmeric, sea salt and ground pepper; gently toss to coat.

Transfer to a baking sheet; bake in the oven for 20 minutes or until Brussels sprouts are tender.

Remove from oven; serve atop a bed of arugula with balsamic vinegar.

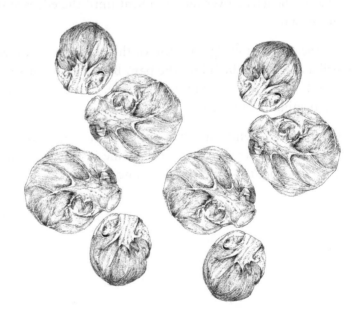

Braised Green Cabbage

—LYDIA GROSSOV—

This quick and easy-to-make dish intensifies the color and brings out the flavor of the green cabbage. It makes for a hearty addition to the main course and a filling, low calorie substitute for starches. It's a surprisingly delicious way to make this mild flavored cruciferous a super star.

Serves 4–6

1 medium (serves 4) or large green cabbage (serves 6)

1 teaspoon extra virgin olive oil

6 medium garlic cloves, thinly sliced

½ teaspoon salt

1 teaspoon fresh ground pepper

½ teaspoon paprika

1 cup of white wine

3 sprigs of fresh or dried thyme

Sit the cabbage stem side down on a cutting board and cut it in half from top to bottom. Cut each half in 2 or 3 wedges (resulting in 4 or 6 wedges) and set aside. *Note:* Leave the stem on the wedges so they won't fall apart.

Place the olive oil and garlic in a large and deep braising pan or frying pan with a lid. Cook the garlic over medium heat until the edges start to sizzle, but do not let them brown.

Place the cabbage wedges on top of the garlic, sprinkle with salt, pepper and paprika and place the lid on the pan. Braise each cut side of the wedges until golden brown, about 2 minutes per side. Make sure to move the garlic around while turning the wedges over.

Place sprigs of thyme into the pan, pour the wine over the wedges and place the lid back on the pan. Cook until the wine is reduced to a thin layer on the bottom of the pan, about 6-8 minutes, turning each wedge over once mid-way through.

Cabbage and Red Apple Slaw

—JILL NUSSINOW—

This recipe takes just a few minutes to make in your food processor. Since cabbage, apples and carrots are almost always available, you can make this anytime, but it's especially refreshing in the winter, when green salad might not seem as appealing, and lettuce can be expensive. It's terrific to bring to potlucks, since you'll be sure to have vegetables to eat.

Serves 6

1½ pounds green cabbage, finely shredded

1 red apple, grated

1 large carrot, grated

1½ tablespoons maple syrup

2–3 tablespoons apple cider vinegar

1 tablespoon Dijon mustard

½ teaspoon sea salt

Quarter the cabbage, remove and discard the central white core. Shred the cabbage by cutting very thin slices along the length of each quarter. You should have about 6 cups. You can use the thin slicing disk of the food processor for this.

Place the shredded cabbage in a large bowl. Toss in the carrots and apple. In a small jar, combine the maple syrup, vinegar, mustard and salt. Shake vigorously and pour over the cabbage. Taste and add more vinegar if desired.

Refrigerate for at least half an hour before serving.

Cabbage Lime Salad
with Dijon-Lime Dressing

—CATHY FISHER—

Using cabbage instead of regular lettuce makes for a hearty salad, perfect served as an entrée. With cabbage and carrots as the foundation, almost any vegetables or beans you have on hand can be added. Sometimes I keep it really simple, using only cabbage, carrots and chickpeas, and other times I just keep adding veggies until it's a rainbow of colors.

Serves 4

SALAD

½ head small-medium green
  cabbage, very thinly sliced
  (about 4 cups), core removed

2 carrots, grated (about 1½ cups)

2 ribs celery, diced

1 red bell pepper, diced

3 green onions/scallions, chopped

½ medium cucumber, peeled
  and diced

¼ cup chopped fresh basil
  (about 20 large leaves)

1½ cups cooked garbanzo or black
  beans or 1 (15-ounce) can

1 avocado, diced

DRESSING

Juice from 2 limes, about ¼ cup

2 tablespoons Dijon mustard

½ teaspoon garlic powder
  (or 1 garlic clove, minced)

For the salad: Using a chef's knife or mandolin slicer, slice the cabbage so that the strands are very thin, and place into a large bowl. Add to this the grated carrots, celery, bell pepper, onion, cucumber, basil, beans, and avocado. Toss.

For the dressing: In a small bowl, combine dressing ingredients and blend with a fork. Add dressing to bowl of vegetables and toss thoroughly. If you are making this ahead of time, add the diced avocado just before serving.

Really Reubenesque Revisited Pizza

—MARK SUTTON—

Here we deconstruct the classic "Reuben Sandwich" and re-formulate the key food elements as a heart healthy, "CHAMPS" dietary contender. The canvas starts with a pumpernickel crust (made with "ancient grain" rye flour, cocoa powder, and caraway seeds), followed by a tangy Thousand Islands Dressing (incorporating tofu, tomato, red wine vinegar, and chopped pickles). The pizza's filling is a crisp mixture of red and green cabbage, mushrooms, and sweet red onions. Roping it all together requires a thick and dynamic fiber-full barley, white bean, and horseradish topping sauce. A nutritional knockout!

Serves 8–12

Pumpernickel or Rye Dough
(recipe below)

Thousand Islands Dressing
(recipe below)

Barley, White Bean, and Horseradish Sauce *(recipe below)*

TOPPING

2 cups (approximately) chopped or sliced red and green cabbage

1 cup (approximately) sliced mushrooms

Sliced onions (as desired)

Preheat oven to 425°F–450°F.

Make the dough. Roll dough out and transfer to baking pan. Spread Thousand Islands Dressing on pizza dough, then arrange topping ingredients as desired. Lastly, gently spread Barley, White Bean, and Horseradish Sauce over the toppings. Bake pizza for 15–20 minutes, depending upon your oven. Let pizza cool a few minutes before slicing and serving.

Pumpernickel or Rye Dough

Surprisingly, molasses is a significant source of iron, calcium, and coper.
It harmonizes brilliantly with rye's high fiber flavor.

1 1/3 to 1 2/3 cups warm water

1 tablespoon oil (optional)

2 tablespoons molasses

1 1/2 cup unbleached whole wheat bread flour

3/4 cup rye flour

2 tablespoons cocoa powder

2 teaspoons instant coffee granules (optional)

1 tablespoon caraway seeds

1 teaspoon salt (optional)

1 1/2 teaspoons active dry yeast

Whisk together warm water, sugar, and yeast and let sit until bubbly for 5 minutes.

Mix together flours and salt in a large bowl. Slowly add this to the yeast mixture (if not using a bread machine on "dough" or "pizza" setting, stir as flour mixture is added).

Knead until the dough is elastic. Put into a bowl and place in a warm pot. Cover with a towel and let rise, covered, for at least an hour until doubled.

Shape pizza dough on a lightly oiled (if desired) non-stick baking sheet or parchment paper on a sheet pan.

Arrange toppings and sauce(s) on top of shaped dough.

Bake in the oven, preheated to 425°F for 15–20 minutes, or until toppings are cooked through.

Notes: To make "rye crust" instead of pumpernickel, omit cocoa flour and coffee granules.

Thousand Islands Dressing Sauce

Quick and easy, this sauce will refrigerate quite nicely for days in a covered container. Stir when ready to use. Chopped seeded cucumbers can substitute for sweet pickles if there's a sugar-related concern.

1 (12.3 ounce) box *Mori-Nu Lite* extra firm tofu

1 tablespoon prepared horseradish (optional)

¼ teaspoon dry mustard

2 tablespoons red wine vinegar

3 tablespoons tomato paste

¼ cup water

½ teaspoon salt

½ cup chopped sweet pickles

If the mixture is too thick, add additonal water, 1 tablespoon at a time, until it's a smoother sauce.

Barley, White Beans, and Horseradish Sauce

More than 1,800 years ago the gladiators of Rome were known as "hordearii" (literally, barley-eaters). They were vegetarians by choice! Preferring to fuel themselves with barley and legumes, they took advantage of the fiber, iron, niacin, and manganese in barley with the protein, fiber, folate, and potassium in beans. This thick and filling topping sauce does, too.

⅓ cup pearl barley

1¼ cups water

1 cup cooked white beans (Cannellini, Great Northern, etc.)

2 tablespoons corn starch

½ tablespoon prepared horseradish

½ tablespoon wet mustard (optional)

¾ cup water

Rinse and drain the beans to remove any salt.

Bring 1¼ cups water and barley to a boil. Cover and turn down the heat to low. Simmer, covered, for 30–40 minutes or less (until the water is absorbed). Let barley cool to room temperature.

Add all ingredients except the water to a blender or food processor, pulse a few times, and add half the water, pulse, and then the remaining water to blend until it's a smooth and thick pancake-like batter.

Note: Makes enough sauce for two 12-inch to 14-inch pizzas (around 3 cups) or one large pizza.

Simple Sauerkraut

—JILL NUSSINOW—

I did not make up this recipe, it is the standard recipe used by Sandor Katz and others, and how it turns out will depend upon many factors, most of which are out of my control, and yours. It may take a few tries before you get it just right but it is worth it. This is a simple fermentation and one that I repeat often with the addition of many different cruciferous vegetables. The possibilities are limited only by your imagination and access to fresh vegetables.

Makes about 1–2 quarts

1 medium to large head cabbage (3–5 pounds)

Pure sea salt, use a scant 2–3 tablespoons for 5 pounds of cabbage and adjust accordingly

Other additions such as garlic, caraway seeds, onion, carrots or more but not too many at once

Remove a large cabbage leaf or two and set aside. Finely slice the cabbage, removing the hard inner core, or cut that very fine. You can do this by hand, which I prefer, or in your food processor or with a mandoline (very carefully). Put the cabbage in a large bowl. Fluff it up and sprinkle the salt on it. Let the cabbage sit with the salt for a few minutes. Then with clean hands and loving intentions, gently massage the cabbage for a few minutes.

Get a very clean (sterilized) half gallon canning jar or other large jar or ceramic vessel, and pack the cabbage mixture into it. As you do this there ought to be liquid appearing in the jar. The goal is to have liquid above the cabbage which will happen if your cabbage is very fresh. Pack the mixture down and put the cabbage leaf on top of it. You can now weigh it down with a rock or glass weights or a plastic bag filled with brine (see what's next).

If you did not get enough liquid from your cabbage, make a brine with 3 tablespoons sea salt to 1 quart of pure (non-chlorinated) water. Heat the water, add the salt and let it cool before adding to your cabbage, only if necessary. Let the cabbage sit for an hour in your jar before adding brine liquid as sometimes the liquid appears.

Cover the jar with a cloth and let sit somewhere around 65°F, protected from animals and insects. If the jar is very full, put it in a bowl as some liquid might come over the edge during fermentation.

Check your mixture daily to be sure that all is OK and that the cabbage is below the liquid. The sauerkraut will be ready to taste starting at a week. You want it to taste sour instead of salty. Most kraut takes a few weeks but a lot depends upon your conditions.

Once your kraut is to your liking, pack into jars and put in the refrigerator. It will last a long time or until you eat it all.

Chipotle Cauliflower Mashers

—ROBIN ROBERTSON—

The smoky heat of chipotle chili gives a flavorful kick to theses mashers made with cauliflower.

Serves 4

- 1 large head cauliflower, trimmed, cored, and coarsely chopped
- 1 or 2 chipotle chilis in adobo sauce, minced
- 1 tablespoon olive oil

- ½ teaspoon salt
- ¼ teaspoon freshly ground black pepper
- 2 tablespoons minced fresh chives or scallions

Steam the cauliflower until soft, 5–7 minutes.

Transfer the steamed cauliflower to a food processor along with the minced chipotle chili, olive oil, salt, and pepper. Purée until smooth and well combined.

Serve hot, sprinkled with chives.

Raw Cauliflower Tabbouleh

—JILL NUSSINOW—

The cauliflower stands in for bulgur wheat in this recipe. If you like, you can also use small broccoli florets in this. If tomatoes or red peppers are in season, feel free to add those, too. (Inspired by a recipe in The Clean Plates Cookbook *by Jared Koch with Jill Silverman Hough)*

Serves 4–6

2–3 lemons

1 pound cauliflower, cut into large bite-size pieces to equal about 3–4 cups

1 large cucumber, halved lengthwise and seeded, cut into small dice

8 kalamata olives, minced

1 cup firm tomatoes, diced

½ to 1 cup chopped Italian parsley

1 tablespoon chopped fresh mint

2 tablespoons extra virgin olive oil (optional)

2 tablespoons toasted pine, or other nuts for garnish

Salt, to taste

Zest the lemons to equal 1 tablespoon of zest. Juice the lemons to equal ¼ cup of lemon juice. Set the zest and juice aside.

Place the cauliflower in the food processor and process to chop into grain-like pieces. Or chop by hand.

Transfer cauliflower to a sieve and let drain, if necessary.

Combine drained cauliflower with other ingredients, except nuts. Add salt, to taste.

Serve, garnished with nuts.

Roasted Cauliflower and Chickpea Curry

—AMBER SHEA CRAWLEY—

This recipe is perfect for weeknight multitasking — you'll prepare the fragrant, garbanzo-bean-packed curry as the cauliflower roasts. When it comes time to stir in the roasted cauliflower at the end, it'll be tender and nutty, nearly melting into the rich, exotic stew. Curry powder is my favorite "shortcut spice;" be sure to shop around and find a blend that you truly love. You can serve the curry over brown rice or quinoa if you want, but it makes a great meal as-is!

Serves 4–6

- 1 medium head cauliflower, stem removed, cut or broken into small florets
- 1 tablespoon good-quality curry powder
- 1/8 teaspoon sea salt
- Vegetable cooking spray
- 1 tablespoons coconut oil (or 2 tablespoons vegetable broth)
- 1 tablespoon cumin seeds
- 2 teaspoons mustard seeds
- 1 large yellow onion, diced

- 2 cloves garlic, peeled and minced
- Small chunk of fresh ginger, peeled and minced
- 2 tablespoons good-quality curry powder
- 1 (28-ounce) can diced tomatoes, partially drained
- 3 cups cooked chickpeas (or 2 (15-ounce) cans, rinsed and drained)
- 2 teaspoons garam masala
- 1–2 teaspoons sea salt, or to taste

Preheat the oven to 400°F (hint: chop your cauliflower while the oven is heating up) and line a rimmed baking sheet with parchment paper or (greased) aluminum foil.

Place the cauliflower in a large bowl. Sprinkle on the curry powder and salt and toss until fairly evenly coated, then spread the cauliflower onto the lined baking sheet in a single layer. Mist the cauliflower lightly all over with cooking spray.

Roast for about 15 minutes, then remove from the oven just long enough to gently toss the mixture around with a spatula or fork.

Return to the oven and roast for 10–15 more minutes, until the cauliflower is fork-tender and golden brown and your kitchen smells nutty and fragrant.

Meanwhile, as the cauliflower is roasting, heat the oil (or broth) in a large pot on the stove over medium heat. Add the cumin and mustard seeds and cover the pot with a lid for about 30 seconds. When you hear the mustard seeds start to pop, take off the lid and add the diced onion. Cook, stirring occasionally, for about 5 minutes, until the onion is softened.

Add the garlic, ginger, and curry powder and cook and stir for 1 more minute.

Stir in the tomatoes and chickpeas, bring to a boil, lower the heat to medium-low, and cook for 5–10 minutes, until slightly thickened.

Add the garam masala and sea salt to taste. Stir in the prepared Curry-Roasted Cauliflower and cook until everything is heated through and the curry has thickened up to your liking.

Roasted Cauliflower
with Arugula Pesto

—ROBIN ROBERTSON—

Roasting gives cauliflower a deep, almost nutty, flavor that is enhanced by the bold arugula pesto.

Serves 4

CAULIFLOWER

1 head cauliflower, trimmed, cored, and cut into ½-inch thick slices

Olive oil or cooking spray

Salt and freshly ground black pepper

PESTO

3 garlic cloves, crushed

¼ cup toasted walnut pieces

½ teaspoon salt

2 cups coarsely chopped arugula

½ cup fresh basil leaves

2 tablespoons olive oil

1 tablespoon lemon juice

¼ teaspoon freshly ground black pepper

Warm water, as needed

For the cauliflower: Preheat the oven to 425°F. Lightly oil a baking sheet or spray it with cooking spray. Arrange the cauliflower slices on the prepared baking sheet. Spray the cauliflower lightly with cooking spray or brush with a little olive oil. Season with salt and pepper to taste. Roast until just tender, 12–14 minutes, turning once halfway through.

For the pesto: While the cauliflower is roasting, make the pesto. In a food processor, combine the garlic, walnuts, and salt and process to a paste. Add the arugula, basil, olive oil, lemon juice, and pepper, and process to a paste. Add a little warm water, if desired, a tablespoon at a time, to reach the desired consistency.

To serve: Remove the cauliflower from the oven and transfer to a shallow serving platter. Serve hot, topped with the pesto.

Collard Green and Quinoa Taco
or Burrito Filling

—KATHY HESTER—

This recipe is one of my favorites because it has a ton of leeway. Have leftover rice or millet? Use it in place of the quinoa. No red peppers? Use green peppers or toss in the leftover cooked veggies from last night. I love collards in this dish but any quick cooking green will do. Your family will never know you're actually cleaning out the fridge on taco night!

Serves 4–6

½ to 1 cup broth or water, divided

½ small onion (about ½ cup)

½ medium red bell pepper (about ½ cup)

3 cloves garlic, minced

1½ cups cooked quinoa

1½ to 2 teaspoons cumin powder, to taste

1½ to 2 teaspoons chili powder, to taste

½ teaspoon smoked paprika

1½ cup chopped collards

¼ cup nutritional yeast flakes

Salt, to taste

Add a few tablespoons of broth or water to a large pan and heat over medium heat. Add onion and sauté until translucent. Add the red pepper, as well as more broth as the pan gets dry. Cook for about 5 minutes more or until the peppers become tender.

Add more broth if the pan is dry so the mixture will not stick to the pan. Stir in the cooked quinoa, 1½ teaspoons cumin powder, 1½ teaspoons chili powder and all the paprika. Cook and stir until the mixture just starts to get rid of the excess liquid. Then stir in the collards and the nutritional yeast.

Cook for 2–3 minutes more or until the collards become tender. Mix in some salt, taste and add more spices if needed. Serve in baked taco shells or whole wheat burrito shells. You can also use soft taco shells or whole wheat and gluten-free choices as needed.

Add toppings such as lettuce, tomatoes, avocado or salsa. If you are avoiding taco or burrito shells, this also makes a tasty and nutritious salad topping!

Collard Greens Wrapped Rolls
with Spiced Quinoa Filling

—JILL NUSSINOW—

You can do this recipe with large leaves of kale or mustard if you don't have collard greens.

Serves 6 main dishes of 2 rolls each

2 tablespoons olive oil, divided

1 cup quinoa, rinsed well

1 cinnamon stick

2 teaspoons curry powder

1¾ cups stock or water

At least 18 large leaves of collard greens, 12 of which must be intact, washed well but not dried

½ cup chopped onion

3 tablespoons toasted pine nuts

¼ cup golden raisins or currants

2 tablespoons lemon juice

Salt and freshly ground black pepper, to taste

2 cups tomato sauce

2 tablespoons golden raisins or currants

Put a medium-sized saucepan on the heat. Add the oil and heat and then add the quinoa and toast. Add cinnamon stick and stock or water; bring to boil. Cover and reduce heat to simmer for 12 minutes. Remove from heat; let stand 5 minutes before uncovering. Remove cinnamon stick.

While the quinoa is cooking, steam or blanch 12 intact collards (or other green) leaves for 2–3 minutes so they will be more pliable. Remove thick stems from steamed leaves; chop stems. Set steamed leaves and chopped stems aside. Remove and discard stems from uncooked collard leaves.

Chop half of the uncooked chard leaves. Heat remaining tablespoon of oil in skillet. Add onion and steamed, chopped stems and sauté over medium heat for 1–2 minutes. Add chopped uncooked leaves, pine nuts and raisins or currants. Cook until collards are wilted, about 3–4 minutes.

Combine quinoa mixture with collard mixture. Add lemon juice; stir well. Season with salt and pepper.

Line a thick-bottomed skillet or pot with remaining uncooked collard leaves. Now gather the 12 intact, blanched leaves. Take one leaf and put ⅓ cup quinoa mixture on bottom third of leaf, stem side toward you. Fold sides of leaf in then roll tightly upward. Put into the leaf-lined skillet or pot. Repeat with remaining steamed leaves.

Mix tomato sauce with 2 tablespoons raisins or currants; pour mixture over stuffed leaves. Cover skillet or pot; cook on low heat 30 minutes. Let the stuffed leaves sit for a few minutes.

Mediterranean Greens

—JILL NUSSINOW—

I find that greens are incredibly versatile. This dish wows people who say that they don't like greens because it has a wonderful mix of sweet, sour and salty. Serve it as appetizer or side dish. Either way it's a winner.

Serves 4–6 as an appetizer served on crackers or 4 as a side dish

1 tablespoon olive oil, optional

½ cup finely minced onion

2 pounds greens, such as collards, kale, mustard, washed but not dried with thick center ribs removed

¼ cup currants or golden raisins

Broth or water, as needed

¼ cup finely chopped Kalamata olives

1 to 2 tablespoons balsamic vinegar

1 tablespoon extra virgin olive oil, optional

Freshly ground black pepper, to taste

Heat the oil in a sauté pan over medium heat, if using. Add the onion and sauté for 3–4 minutes until it turns translucent. Add the greens and sauté for 1 minute. Add the currants or raisins until the greens turn bright green. Stir in the olives.

If greens get dry during cooking, add broth or water, 1 tablespoon at a time, being careful not to let the mixture get too liquid. Remove from the heat and let cool a bit. Add the vinegar and oil, if using. Add pepper to taste.

Smoky Collard Greens

—MORGAN ECCLESTON—

This is a classic collard green dish that goes perfectly with a batch of cornbread to soak up the pot liquor (the broth) and some black-eyed peas for good measure.

Serves 4–6

2 large bunch collard greens, stems removed and chopped

1 large onion, chopped

3 cloves garlic, minced

5 cups vegetable broth

½ teaspoon kosher salt

½–1 teaspoon chipotle powder

½ teaspoons apple cider vinegar

Sauté the chopped onion with 2 tablespoons of water in a large pot over high heat until translucent. Add in the garlic and cook one minute longer or until fragrant.

Add collard greens, broth, salt and chipotle powder. Bring to a boil and turn the heat to low and cover. Simmer for 45 minutes or until the greens are super tender.

Add in the vinegar to taste.

Horseradish and Cannellini Bean Dip

—BEVERLY BENNETT—

Prepared horseradish adds a pungent "zing" to this fat-free dip. You can serve this tasty dip with an assortment of raw veggies, crackers, flatbreads, or small slices of toasted bread, and it can also be used as a spread for sandwiches or wraps.

Serves: 4 (¼ cup) servings or 2 cups

1 (15-ounce) can cannellini beans, drained and rinsed

¼ cup prepared horseradish

3 tablespoons water

1 tablespoon nutritional yeast flakes

In a food processor fitted with an S blade, combine the cannellini beans, horseradish, water, and nutritional yeast flakes and process for 1–2 minutes or until smooth. Scrape down the sides of the container with a spatula and process for an additional 15 seconds.

Transfer the dip to an airtight container. Serve immediately with raw veggies, crackers or bread slices as desired. Store in an airtight container in the refrigerator for up to 3–4 days.

Variations: For a milder flavored dip, only add 2–3 tablespoons prepared horseradish. You can also prepare this dip with other varieties of white beans, such as navy, white kidney, or great Northern.

Kale-Apple Slaw
with Goji Berry Dressing

—J.L. FIELDS—

The blend of goji berries with apples and carrots makes a distinct slaw that's sure to impress.

Serves 4

SALAD

1 large apple, cored and quartered (no need to peel)

2 large carrots

1 large stalk of celery

3 curly kale leaves (with stems)

DRESSING

1 tablespoon avocado oil (or extra virgin olive oil)

2 tablespoons apple cider vinegar

1 teaspoon whole grain mustard

¼ cup filtered water

1 clove garlic

¼ cup dried Goji berries (or other dried, unsulphured fruit, such as raisins, currants, cranberries, or mulberries)

Ground black pepper, to taste

Shred the apple, carrots, celery and kale in a food processor (use the slicing blade) or on a mandoline slicer. Transfer to a large bowl.

Blend all dressing ingredients in a blender or food processor. Pour dressing over the shredded ingredients and toss.

Store in an airtight container and refrigerate for at least 30 minutes.

Hail to the Kale Salad

—CHEF AJ—

Even people who say that don't like kale will gobble this up.

Serves 4–6

DRESSING

1 cup raw almond butter (unsweetened and unsalted)

1 cup coconut, or regular, water

¼ cup fresh lime juice (about 2 limes) plus ¼ teaspoon lime zest

2 cloves garlic

1-inch or ½ ounce (approximate) fresh, peeled ginger

2 tablespoons low sodium tamari or raw coconut aminos

4 pitted Medjool dates (soaked in water if not soft)

½ teaspoon red pepper flakes

SALAD

2 large heads of curly kale (about 24 ounces) finely chopped with thick stems removed

½ cup chopped almonds

In a high powered blender combine all dressing ingredients until smooth and creamy.

Remove the thick, larger stems from the kale, finely chop and place in a large bowl. Pour the dressing over the kale and massage the dressing into the kale while using your hands. Sprinkle with almonds before serving. Like a woman, this only gets better with age.

Chef's Note: This salad is also delicious when made with peanut butter or tahini or when you add some shredded raw beets and carrots to the salad. If you have a dehydrator, dip kale leaves in the dressing and dehydrate for delicious kale chips!

Kid's Kale

—TESS CHALLIS—

When children first see this, they often proclaim that they will have nothing to do with it. However, when they finally try it, they invariably scarf it down and ask for seconds! You can feel like a champion eating this, as kale is one of the most immune boosting, energizing, and strengthening vegetables around. It is also ridiculously high in calcium, iron, and vitamins. Admittedly, I belong to the elitist cult that prefers the lacinato variety (also called black kale).

Serves 4

1 pound (4 cups packed) lacinato kale ribbons, washed well

¼ cup liquid vegetarian broth

2 teaspoons oil (coconut, olive, or sunflower)

4 medium cloves garlic, minced or pressed

4 teaspoons tamari, shoyu, or soy sauce

4 teaspoons fresh lemon juice

2 teaspoons nutritional yeast powder

Place the kale on a cutting board and cut off the thickest portion of the stem base. I don't remove the stems above this point, as they are tender enough to eat when cooked (if finely chopped). Cut the kale into thin ribbons.

Place the kale along with the broth, oil, garlic, and tamari into a medium-large skillet. Cook over medium-high heat for about 5 minutes, stirring often, until bright green. Remove from heat. Toss with two teaspoons of the lemon juice and the nutritional yeast powder.

The Veggie Queen's Husband's Daily Green Smoothie

—JILL NUSSINOW—

I make this daily. It can be made with kale, collards or your favorite green although it's not especially tasty to my husband with anything bitter like arugula. I soak the nuts overnight, drain and store in the refrigerator for the week. I also rehydrate the chia weekly by combining 3 tablespoons chia seed with 1 cup water and mixing well.

Serves 1 large smoothie

5 soaked almonds

2 tablespoons rehydrated chia

1 cup packed kale, stems included

1 cup frozen fruit, seasonal when you can

1 cup frozen berries

½ medium banana

1 cup water

Blend in a high speed blender until smooth and creamy. Serve right away.

If you have any leftover, put into ice cube trays to make "smoothie cubes" and blend later.

The Veggie Queen's Raw Kale Salad

—JILL NUSSINOW—

This is easy to make and you'll get a great dose of greens. Use your favorites types, put in extras to suit your taste. The only limit to what goes into this salad is your imagination. When you massage the greens, be sure to add the love.

Serves 2–4

- 1–2 bunches kale, collards or other greens, washed and spun dry
- 2–3 teaspoons raw tahini
- 1 tablespoon lemon juice
- 1–2 teaspoons miso (my favorite is *South River Miso*—brown rice or mellow white works well) or *Bragg Liquid Aminos*
- 1 teaspoon agave, or more to taste or soaked, blended dates
- 1 apple or pear, sliced thin, julienned or grated
- ½ avocado, cut into chunks, if you like it
- Top with seeds, if desired

Remove leaves from large ribs and slice thinly. Put into a large bowl. Add the tahini, lemon juice and miso. Put your hands into the bowl and massage the greens until they are wilted, about 3–5 minutes. Add the agave or date syrup and apple or pear and avocado. Stir well to combine. This tastes best when eaten immediately.

Notice how the greens shrink by about half when they are massaged with the tahini, miso and lemon juice. If you are eating this by yourself, make half a batch at once.

Note: You can also add sunflower seeds or dried fruit to this salad, or go more savory by adding crushed garlic and sliced onion and omitting the apple.

Crunchy Kohlrabi Quinoa Salad

—MARY MCDOUGALL—

This delicious salad is easy to put together and stays fresh tasting and crunchy while it is chilling in the refrigerator. It can easily be modified using whatever vegetables you have in your garden or have found at the farmers' market.

Preparation Time: 30 minutes
Chilling Time: 1–2 hours

Serves 6

1 cup uncooked quinoa, well rinsed

2 cups vegetable broth

3 2-inch strips of lemon zest

1½ cups asparagus, sliced into ½-inch pieces

1 cup snow peas, cut in half

½ cup kohlrabi, peeled and sliced into thin strips

⅓ cup radishes, thinly sliced

3 tablespoons lemon juice

2 tablespoons chopped fresh chives

2 tablespoons chopped fresh parsley

1 tablespoon chopped fresh cilantro (optional)

1 teaspoon chopped fresh mint

Freshly ground pepper

Dash sea salt

Place quinoa in a pot with the vegetable broth and bring to a boil. Reduce heat, stir in the pieces of lemon zest, cover and cook for 15 minutes. Remove from heat, stir, remove pieces of lemon zest (discard) and let quinoa cool slightly.

Meanwhile, put a large pot of water on to boil, drop in asparagus and snow peas and cook for 2–3 minutes until crisp-tender. Remove from pot with tongs and drop into a bowl of ice water. Drain.

Combine quinoa, asparagus, snow peas, kohlrabi and radishes in a large bowl. Add remaining ingredients and mix well. Season with freshly ground pepper and sea salt, if desired. Chill for 1–2 hours before serving to allow flavors to mingle.

Hints: Wash the lemon and then peel with a vegetable peeler, yielding very thin strips. Use the remaining lemon for the juice in this recipe. Kohlrabi may be unfamiliar to you, but I highly recommend it in this recipe. Look for it in farmers' markets or in large supermarkets or natural food stores. If you can't find it, you may just omit it, or use fresh zucchini or cucumber instead.

Balsamic Glazed Herb Roasted Roots
with Kohlrabi, Rutabaga, Turnip, Fennel, Carrots and Potatoes

—JILL NUSSINOW—

I love roasted roots. I am not a big fennel fan but it takes on a wonderful mellow flavor when roasted. To roast well, the vegetables need a lot of space and far less oil than you think. The addition of herbs boosts the flavor. When cutting the vegetables, work on making the pieces of similar size so that they cook evenly.

Serves 4–6

2 onions, cut into halves or quarters

10 cloves garlic, unpeeled

1–2 medium kohlrabi, peeled and cubed to equal 2–3 cups

1 medium rutabaga, peeled and cubes to equal 2 cups

4–6 small to medium turnips, tops removed and cut in half or quarters to equal at least 1 cup of similar size as other vegetables

1 medium fennel bulb, fronds removed, sliced thin

2 cups carrots, peeled and cut into 1 to 2-inch pieces

6–8 fingerling or other small potatoes, cut into 1½ inch pieces

2 tablespoons olive oil

Salt and pepper

3 sprigs rosemary

3 sprigs thyme

GLAZE

2 tablespoons neutral oil, optional

3 tablespoons maple syrup

2 tablespoons balsamic vinegar

½ teaspoon chopped fresh or dried rosemary

Preheat the oven to 425°F. Combine all the vegetables in a large glass baking dish or two. Add the olive oil, salt and pepper and toss well. Add the herb sprigs. Cover the dish. Bake for 30 minutes.

Remove the cover and see if the vegetables are cooked through. Cook, uncovered, for another 5 minutes or until the vegetables are tender but not mushy.

You can also do this on open sheet pans with lots of space around the vegetables. Covering the vegetables allows them to steam a bit which allows you to use much less oil without a loss of flavor.

While the vegetables are cooking, combine the glaze ingredients and cook for about 5–10 minutes until thickened and syrupy. Pour over the vegetables right before serving and stir to combine. Serve hot on a large platter.

Mustard Greens and Gumbo

—JASON WYRICK—

This recipe is actually three parts. You've got the gumbo, the rice, and the garlicky mustard greens, each of which is served in a way to distinguish the three components. This gives the recipe an added layer of complexity in taste than it would if everything was simply mixed together. Also, I like my food very spicy, so feel free to modify the amount of cayenne used in the recipe.

Serves 2

GUMBO

1 small sweet onion, diced
½ green bell pepper, diced
1 stalk of celery, diced
2 cloves of garlic, minced
¼ cup whole wheat pastry flour
2 cups veggie broth
½ cup sliced okra
½ teaspoon salt
¼ teaspoon cayenne
1 teaspoon fresh thyme
2 bay leaves
Hot sauce to taste

GARLICKY MUSTARD GREENS

1 large bunch mustard greens, sliced
  (including the ribs)
4 cloves garlic, minced
Pinch of salt
¼ cup water

RICE

½ cup long grain brown rice
Pinch of salt and black pepper

Dice the onion, bell pepper, and celery and mince the garlic. In a dry pot over a medium heat, toast the flour for about 2 minutes. Add the onion, bell pepper, celery, and garlic (do not add any liquid!), and sauté this until the onion just starts to brown, stirring slowly the whole time.

Add the veggie broth, okra, salt, cayenne, thyme, and bay leaves. Reduce the heat to medium low and simmer this for at least 10 minutes. You should have a semi-thick sauce when you are done. If the sauce thickens to the point where there isn't much sauce left at all, add in ½ cup of veggie broth at the end, and stir.

Slice the garlic greens and mince the garlic. In a dry pan over a medium heat, sauté the garlic for 2 minutes. Add the water, then the greens and salt and cook until the greens are completely wilted and the ribs are soft.

Cook the rice according to your preferred method, adding in the salt and pepper at the beginning of the cooking process.

Mound the rice in the plate, pour the gumbo over it, top with the greens, and serve with hot sauce.

Time Management Tip: Start the rice before you start working on the gumbo and they should both be done about the same time. You can also cook the greens while the gumbo is simmering, since you won't much need to pay attention to the gumbo at that point.

Mustard Greens, Snow Peas, Green Garlic and Kumquats Spring Slaw

—JILL NUSSINOW—

This crisp salad is based on what is fresh in the garden, market or what's in your refrigerator. Optional ingredients are shredded fennel, kohlrabi or Jerusalem artichoke. This s an alternative to green salad or feel free to eat both. Few people get too many vegetables.

Serves 4 to 6

2 cups assorted mustard greens, sliced thin

6 cups Napa or other cabbage, sliced thin

½ teaspoon salt

1–2 stalks green garlic, minced

2 cups sliced snow or sugar snap peas

2 green onions, sliced

½ cup sliced kumquats

1 orange, juiced

2 teaspoons rice vinegar

Combine the mustard greens and cabbage with the salt and toss. Let sit for at least 15 minutes, then squeeze to extract liquid.

Combine with the remaining ingredients and chill. Serve chilled or at room temperature. Best eaten within a couple of hours of making it.

Cinnamon Roasted Radishes

—AMIE VALPONE—

A very non-traditional way to use radishes. This is very simple to prepare and deceptively divine.

Serves 2

1 bunch red radishes, leaves remove

2 tablespoons coconut oil

1 teaspoon fresh lemon juice

¼ teaspoon ground ginger

¼ teaspoon ground cinnamon

¼ teaspoon sea salt

¼ teaspoon freshly ground pepper

Preheat oven to 350°F. In a large bowl, combine radishes with remaining ingredients; gently toss to combine.

Transfer to a baking sheet; bake for 25 minutes or until radishes are tender.

Remove from oven; serve warm.

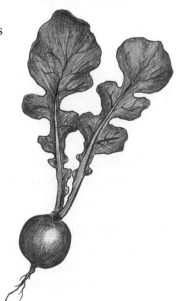

Daikon Radish Rawvioli
with Creamy Nut filling

—JILL NUSSINOW—

This is easy to make when root vegetables are around that can be sliced thinly on the mandolin. That is part of the key to making this tasty dish. It is time consuming so only make it for those who will appreciate it wholeheartedly.

Serves 4

1 medium watermelon or other daikon, kohlrabi or turnip that can be sliced thinly on a mandoline

FILLING

¼ cup fresh lemon juice

¼ cup water

2 cloves garlic

1 cup raw cashews, macadamia nuts, pine nuts or a combination

¼ to ½ teaspoon salt

Chopped fresh herbs, if desired

For the filling: Process in a high speed blender until smooth and creamy. It should be quite thick. Taste to be sure that you don't have to adjust the seasonings — it should be savory.

To assemble: To make the rawvioli, put down a slice of the root vegetable, put a teaspoon of the filing inside and fold the vegetable in half to seal shut or for a harder vegetable, put two together. It's okay if some of the filling squeezes out. Chill, if not serving right away.

Mango, Daikon, and Avocado Spring Rolls

—MIYOKO SCHINNER—

This delicious spring roll is not the typical kind filled with raw veggies, dipped in peanut sauce. This one tickles your palate with its light and refreshing combination of sweet, tangy, citrusy, and salty. The creamy mango and avocado offset the cool, crispness of raw daikon radish. For parties, I always like to serve a combination of lighter and richer appetizers, and this is one of my "go to" light appetizers.

Serves 8–10

6 ounces daikon, peeled and julienned

1 large mango, peeled and julienned

½ an English cucumber, peeled and julienned

1 large avocado, peeled and cut into strips

8–10 rice paper rounds

Bowl of hot water for dipping

To make the spring rolls, one piece at a time, dip the rice paper in the hot water for 5–10 seconds to soften. Put the rice paper on a clean surface. Working quickly, place a small and equal amount of the daikon, mango, avocado, and cucumber on the rice paper on the end closest to you. Fold in the sides, then roll as tightly as possible. Cut each into 4–6 pieces.

Root Veggies Paté

—KAREN RANZI—

It's hard to believe that such a simple combination of vegetables can produce such spectacular results. And it's so easy to prepare.

Serves 2–4

3 medium carrots, chopped

1 stalk celery, chopped

1 medium rutabaga, peeled and chopped

Juice of ½ lemon

Juice of ½ lime

2 tablespoons raw tahini

Process carrots, celery and rutabaga in food processor until finely ground. Add lemon and lime juice and tahini and process until a smooth paté. This is one of my favorite dishes to place over a large green salad for a complete meal.

Rutabaga "Noodles"
with Lemon Balsamic Tahini Sauce

—HEATHER NICHOLDS—

This is a very simple raw noodle dish with a light lemon dressing, and is perfect for a night when you want a light but nourishing meal. You can cook the rutabaga if you prefer, but it's incredibly delicious eaten raw once it's spiralized or grated. Raw vegetables retain all of their natural nutrients and enzymes, and are nice and cooling for a hot summer evening.

Serves 4–6

2 large rutabaga, spiralized or grated

Pinch sea salt

DRESSING

1 lemon, zested and juiced

4 tablespoons tahini

2 tablespoons balsamic vinegar

1–2 cloves garlic, pressed

Sea salt, to taste

½ cup fresh parsley, chopped

½ cup fresh mint, chopped

3 green onions, chopped

½ cup olives, pitted and chopped

Process the rutabaga through a spiralizer, to make into thin noodles, or you can grate it if you don't have a spiralizer. I like to use my food processor's grating blade for this, because it's so fast and it also makes a thicker grate. Don't use a fine grater, otherwise your rutabaga will be too mushy. Put the spiralized or grated rutabaga in a large bowl, sprinkle with a pinch of sea salt and toss. Leave it to marinate while you prepare the dressing.

For the dressing: First zest the lemon, then squeeze the juice in a small bowl or jar and whisk it together with the tahini and balsamic vinegar. Add a bit of water to adjust the consistency. Mix in the lemon zest, pressed garlic and just enough sea salt to bring the flavors together.

Next, chop up the fresh herbs and olives, and toss them together. I like to serve the rutabaga noodles topped with the fresh herb mixture and then drizzled with dressing. You can also toss the rutabaga "noodles" with the dressing to coat them and then serve sprinkled with the fresh herb mixture.

Tatsoi with Bok Choy and Mushrooms

—JILL NUSSINOW—

This simple dish also works if you add tofu or tempeh, or your favorite cooked bean. In many recipes, tatsoi and bok choy are interchangeable.

Serves 4

- 2 green onions, sliced on the diagonal
- 1 cup sliced crimini, or other, mushrooms
- 2 teaspoons minced ginger
- 2 cloves garlic, minced
- 2 cups tatsoi, chopped

- 4 baby bok choy to equal about 3 cups chopped
- 2 teaspoons tamari
- ¼ cup vegetable broth
- Toasted sesame seeds, or hemp seeds for garnish

Heat a large sauté pan over medium heat. Add the green onions and mushrooms and dry sauté for a minute or two. Add the ginger and garlic and sauté one more minute, adding some of the broth if things start to stick.

Add the tatsoi, bok choy, tamari and the rest of the vegetable broth. Simmer for 3–4 minutes until the mushrooms are cooked through and the greens are bright green.

Serve hot, garnished with sesame or hemp seeds.

Braised Turnip Greens
with Tomatoes and Thyme

—JILL NUSSINOW—

When you find young and beautiful turnips, take off their greens right away and use them soon. You can add the tender turnips to this dish, if you like but let the greens be the star. Serve as a side dish or over noodles, quinoa or other grain such as farro, rye, oats or barley.

Serves 4

6 cups chopped turnip greens

1½ cups peeled, seeded, diced tomatoes, fresh or canned

½ cup red wine

1 teaspoon sugar, *Sucanat* or agave syrup

3 cloves garlic, minced

1–2 sprigs fresh thyme or 1 teaspoon dried thyme

1 cinnamon stick

2 tablespoons fruity olive oil (optional)

Combine all ingredients in a non-reactive saucepan over medium heat. Simmer, covered for 15 minutes. Simmer for 15 minutes more, or longer to reduce the mixture to the thickness that you like. Remove the cinnamon stick and thyme branches.

Moroccan Vegetable Tagine

—ELLEN KANNER—

Cumin and cinnamon, the warming traditional flavors of Morocco, shine through in this vegetable tagine (Moroccan stew) without the usual long, slow simmering. This recipe embraces every bit of turnip, from bulb to greens. Serve over quinoa or whole grain couscous.

Serves 4–6

1 tablespoon olive oil

1 onion, sliced

1 bunch young turnips and greens, chopped into bite-sized pieces

2 carrots, chopped

2 stalks celery, chopped

2 peppers, red or green, sliced into strips

1 pound fresh tomatoes, diced or 1 (15-ounce) can organic diced tomatoes

½ teaspoon paprika

½ teaspoon cumin

½ teaspoon cinnamon

1 pinch red pepper flakes

a few saffron threads

1 preserved lemon* chopped fine or juice of 1 fresh lemon

sea salt to taste

1 handful cilantro, chopped

1 handful Italian parsley, chopped

In a large pot, heat the oil over medium-high heat. Add onion, carrot, celery, peppers and turnips and cook, stirring occasionally, until vegetables soften and become fragrant, about 8–10 minutes.

Add paprika, cumin, cinnamon, pepper and saffron. Gently stir in the chopped turnip greens and cook until they start to wilt, another few minutes. Add diced tomatoes and stir to combine.

Bring to boil, then cover and reduce heat to low. Let tagine simmer on its own for 30 minutes or so, until vegetables are tender.

Add chopped preserved lemon or fresh lemon juice. Add sea salt to taste.

Just before serving, stir in chopped parsley and cilantro.

---

*Tangy, salty preserved lemons appear in many Moroccan recipes and are available at Middle Eastern and gourmet food stores.

Scalloped Turnips Casserole

—BEVERLY BENNETT—

Thin slices of turnips and sliced green onions are layered in a creamy sauce and covered with a bread crumb topping to create this comfort food-style side dish, which will turn even the pickiest eaters into turnip lovers.

Serves 6

Oil of choice or cooking spray

2 cups soy or other non-dairy milk

2 tablespoons nutritional yeast flakes

1½ tablespoon garlic powder

2 pounds turnips, peeled, cut in half lengthwise, and thinly sliced

¼ cup thinly sliced green onions (white and green parts)

¼ cup chopped fresh parsley

Sea salt

Freshly ground black pepper

⅓ cup fresh or dried bread crumbs

Smoked or sweet paprika

Preheat the oven to 375°F. Lightly oil (or spray with cooking spray) a 9-inch baking pan or 1½-quart or larger casserole dish.

In a small bowl or measuring cup, whisk together the soy milk, nutritional yeast flakes, and garlic powder, and set aside.

In the prepared baking pan, layer half of the sliced turnips, 2 tablespoons sliced green onions, and 2 tablespoons chopped parsley. Season with salt and pepper to taste. Repeat the layering procedure and season with salt and pepper again.

Pour the soy milk mixture over the top and shake the pan gently to allow some of it to disperse between the layered ingredients. Sprinkle the breadcrumbs and a little paprika over the top for added color and flavor. Bake for 45–50 minutes or until the turnips are fork-tender. Remove from the oven. Serve hot.

Variation: You can also prepare this recipe with 2 pounds parsnips or rutabagas, peeled and thinly sliced, or with a combination of other root vegetables.

Potato and Watercress Soup
with Sorrel Cream

—JILL NUSSINOW—

I never had potato soup that I didn't like. The additional ingredients are perfect for spring as you get the bitter from the watercress and the sour from the sorrel which are useful for "spring cleaning" your body. The soup is creamy and refreshing.

Serves 4-6

SOUP

1 tablespoon olive oil, optional

1 medium onion, diced

2 leeks, cleaned and cut into small pieces

1½ pounds Yukon gold or yellow Finn potatoes, peeled and cut into small dice

4 cups vegetable stock or water

1–2 teaspoons salt (only if using water)

2 cups chopped watercress, thick stems removed

1 cup chopped sorrel

Fresh ground pepper

¼ cup fresh dill

CREAM

1 (12.3 ounce) package *Mori-Nu Lite* firm or extra firm silken tofu

1 tablespoon fresh lemon juice

1 tablespoon canola or olive oil, optional

2 teaspoons rice vinegar

¼ teaspoon salt

1 cup chopped sorrel

Heat the oil in a medium pot over medium heat. Add the onions and leeks and sauté for about 8 minutes, until they start to soften. Add the potatoes and stock and bring to a boil. Reduce the heat to a simmer. (If using water, add salt now.) Simmer for 20 minutes, or until the potatoes are tender.

Remove the pot from the heat. Purée a bit with a hand (immersion) blender, until it reaches the consistency that you desire. Stir in the watercress, sorrel and pepper. Taste and add more salt if desired. Stir in the dill. Top with the sorrel cream.

While the soup is cooking, make the "cream" by placing all the ingredients for the cream except the sorrel into the food processor. Process until smooth. Taste and adjust seasonings. Pulse in the sorrel. Chill for a bit, up to a day. Drizzle over the hot soup.

Watercress-Sage Pesto

—KAMI MCBRIDE—

Depending on how spicy you like your pesto, you can go with one clove of garlic or add more. You can also create some variation to the recipe and add one tablespoon dried tomatoes or one tomatillo. In my house pesto is a garnish for breakfast, lunch and dinner. What a yummy way to get in a serving or two of your greens!

Serves 4

2 cups watercress

1 cup parsley

¼ cup fresh garden sage

¼ cup olive oil

¼ cup sunflower seeds

1–2 garlic cloves

¼ teaspoon salt

1 teaspoon lemon juice

Put watercress, sage, salt and olive oil in a food processor and blend well. Add remaining ingredients until creamy.

Sweet Watercress Smoothie

—CARRIE FORREST—

Watercress tops the list of most nutritious vegetables on the planet, but many people find it too bitter to eat plain. This smoothie uses frozen fruit to mask the flavor of the watercress and the soy milk and almond butter make it creamy and decadent. By adding carob or cacao powder, there is even a hint of chocolate in this refreshing and healthy smoothie.

Serves 2

2 cups unsweetened soy milk

2 tablespoons unsalted almond butter

1 bunch watercress, washed

1 frozen banana

½ cup frozen blackberries or blueberries

1 cup frozen strawberries

1 cup frozen pineapple

1 tablespoon flax meal

1 tablespoon chia seeds

1 tablespoon carob or cacao powder

Add the ingredients to a high-speed blender and process until smooth.

The Great Oil Debate
in which I Refuse to Participate

I have been teaching cooking for more than 25 years. For the past 13 years I have been teaching for Dr. John McDougall who recommends a no-oil added vegan diet. I have experience playing on both sides of the fence. I refuse to debate the subject and since I write books for a general audience who is interested in eating more healthfully, you will often find optional oil in my recipes. You can omit it if you don't want to use it.

You likely know that most people use oil in cooking. If you don't use it, you are in a small, no make that teeny, minority. I am not going to tell you what to do and that you must include any oil. In fact, I have described how to dry sauté as a technique for eliminating oil in cooking (see the "Dry Sautéing" article on page 128).

For me, as a cooking teacher for the general population, I use oil because it makes cooking easier and it's what most people expect. I encourage people to cut their oil use and consumption. Do I think that including a couple of teaspoons or a tablespoon of oil in your food every few days will kill you? I do not. I think that choosing the best-for-you foods most of the time is the key to good health.

I want to point out some interesting facts about oil just because…

In biblical times, certain high priests, and others, were anointed with holy oil which was likely olive oil. The entire Hanukkah story is based on oil and latkes are the poster child for this Jewish holiday. They are always fried and the oil was a source of light.

In ancient times oil was processed on a stone mill. There was no high heat processing and extraction. Oil was fresh and had to be used in a reasonable period of time or it would get rancid. Oil is supposed to get rancid, just the way food is supposed to spoil after a certain amount of time. It's natural for this to occur.

It is noted in the Book of Genesis that when God visited Adam in the Garden of Eden, he gave him the gift of an olive tree to be planted there. God gave precise directions on how to care for the tree in order to produce "oil which would heal man's wounds and cure all ills."

Homer, author of The Iliad and The Odyssey referred to olive oil as "liquid gold."

Hippocrates, the father of modern medicine, studied the benefits of olive oil and suggested its use to cure many diseases. The therapeutic effect was known as far back as 1550 B.C.

What's gone wrong? The world has changed, the food has changed and even the oil has changed but how much have we changed?

We used to need the calories in oil to sustain us but now we have 24-hour supermarkets and food always at our disposal. Oil is not as important in our diets as it was thousands of years ago. In fact it might be downright harmful.

I've been a dietitian for more than thirty years, I have seen many different attempts to solve the "oil crisis." When I was training to be an R.D., the American Heart Association recommendation for combatting heart disease was to include more polyunsaturated oils such as corn, soybean and safflower to lower cholesterol. Then scientists came to realize that those oils caused oxidation and were potentially linked to a higher incidence of cancer.

We changed that recommendation to include more monounsaturated oils such as olive, canola, avocado and macadamia which are less likely to get rancid because of their fatty acid composition.

People (at least here in the U.S.) went olive oil crazy. I am not sure that they have stopped. Some people were even going so far as to drink their oil at the end of the day if they hadn't consumed two tablespoons.

Next we realized (and I always had) that trans fats are not good for you. When you take a fat and change it in an unnatural way through better technology, it's just not beneficial to humans. Mother Nature has a plan and I believe that hers is better than ours. (Just take a look at what we have done to our environment.) This may be the best fat news we've had: get the trans fats out of foods. And avoid the foods that contain partially hyrdrogenated fats, which are mostly found in processed foods. Eat "real" food in its whole form and you don't find trans fats.

This leads us to two other types of fat: coconut oil, which is a very saturated fat, and Omega-3 fatty acids which are super polyunsaturated essential fats.

Now people are cuckoo for coconut oil. Coconut oil contains medium chain triglycerides. I have known since graduate school that these fats behave differently in your body. At that time I did not recommend coconut oil and I still don't recommend it for most people. Most of us live in temperate climates. Coconut oil comes from tropical regions. People have always used the fat of their region because that is what they had.

In the tropics, coconut oil is not hard as a rock, it is liquid or semi-liquid. I cannot see how adding copious amounts of coconut oil to the diet can be good for you (but I could be wrong). Most people do not need the calories. One tablespoon of oil is 120 calories.

Regarding Omega-3 fatty acids, they are fragile and oxidize easily. You can buy flax and hemp oil but it must be stored in the refrigerator to stay fresh. I can guarantee you that people have only had refrigerators as they are now for 100 years and that these oils did not exist before then, or really even 50 years ago. Why didn't we need these essential oils? Obviously we did. They are essential. We must have been eating them.

At some point the ratio between our Omega-3, 6 and 9 fatty acids got out of whack. Possibly it was when we started having more and more processed food in our diet; the types of food that have grown exponentially over the past fifty years. Other than flax, chia and hemp seeds, walnuts, greens and purslane are good plant sources of Omega-3 fatty acids. So cutting back on the vegetable oils and including more of the sources of the essential Omega-3 fatty acids is a good idea. Those seeds still oxidize quickly so use care with them. Keep them whole and grind them when you need them. Or keep them in the refrigerator or freezer. Include them in your diet daily for improved immune function.

If you have heart disease, I highly recommend avoiding all oil and including sources of Omega-3 fatty acids as ground seeds and paying strict attention to what you eat. I will tell you that I know few people who are eating too many greens. Once you think that you are in that camp, come talk to me and we can discuss oil.

—Jill Nussinow

C
H
A
M
P
S

Herbs and Spices Included

Basil

Cayenne

Cilantro

Cinnamon

Cumin

Ginger

Mint

Mustard

Oregano

Parsley

Thyme

Turmeric

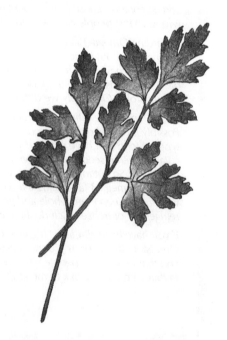

CHAPTER 2

Herbs and Spices

L IKE AN ARTIST with a color palette, using herbs and spices perks up your food, adding bright spots and bold flavors on which to focus your attention. You can elevate a bowl of beans from ordinary to out of this world with just a few shakes of the bottles from your spice cabinet.

If you think back to the time that you learned about the explorers such as Vasco De Gama and Ferdinand Magellan, you might recall that they went halfway around the world to find these products which were considered as valuable as treasure. A pound of nutmeg could be traded for seven fat oxen.

Herbs and spices were certainly culinary treasure as there was no refrigeration then. Spices and herbs not only made the food palatable but it is extremely likely that the high antioxidant activity of spices and herbs kept the food from spoiling as quickly. This was extremely important then and it still is as we need those antioxidants to keep us in great health.

Since these plant foods are highly concentrated, I recommend buying organic herbs and spices whenever possible. In fact, *McCormick,* the huge spice company, has a chart that shows the following antioxidants equivalents:

1 teaspoon ground cinnamon = ½ cup blueberries
½ teaspoon oregano = 3 cups fresh spinach
1 teaspoon curry powder = ½ cup red grapes[1]

An Herb or Spice?

The difference between herbs and spices is which part of the plant you are using. Spices are the seasonings for food that come from the bark, buds, fruit or flower parts, roots, seeds or stems of various aromatic plants and trees. Herbs are the leafy parts of woody, and other, plants.

If you are just entering the world of herbs and spices, I realize that how to use them can often be overwhelming. I will shed some light on this here.

When a recipe calls for fresh herbs and you only have dried use one-third the amount. For example, a recipe calls for 1 tablespoon parsley, use 1 teaspoon dried (there are

[1] *Oxygen Radical Absorbance Capacity* (ORAC) of Selected Foods 2007, Nutrient Data Laboratory USDA, November 2007, http://www.ars.usda.gov/nutrientdata/ORAC

3 teaspoons in a tablespoon). Dried herbs that are especially strong are rosemary, sage, thyme and oregano so feel free to use less and add more herbs later on in cooking. Dried herbs function best when added during cooking and fresh herbs often are added after food has been cooked or at the very end of cooking to preserve their flavor.

Spices often are added during cooking so that they can be absorbed into your dish. Some whole spices such as cumin, coriander and mustard benefit from toasting and grinding to produce more complex and deeper flavors in your food.

Toast the spices in a dry pan over medium heat. Shake the pan and keep the spices moving for a few minutes until they smell toasty and fragrant. Let them cool and then add to your spice grinder (coffee grinder that's not for coffee) until they are ground. Or you can use a mortar and pestle to pulverize them. Do each spice separately for the best flavor. You can clean the oils out of your spice grinder by whirring white rice in it until it is powder. Store the toasted spice in a labeled airtight jar for up to 6 months. (Hopefully you will use them up long before then.)

Purchasing:

To maximize your money and efficiency, if you have availability, purchase your spices and herbs in bulk. You can check out the aromas of the herbs and spices to see which appeal to you. You can buy just a small amount to use in your cooking to see if you like it. It is much less expensive to buy in bulk than in small pre-packaged jars. You can often save fifty percent or more by buying in bulk and you can buy only what you will use in a reasonable period of time. Most dried herbs and ground spices will last six months. When the herbs have lost their aroma when crushed between your fingers, it is time to toss them. When the spices smell dusty or musty, they need to go too. Most dried seeds will last a year or more, unground, but if they smell at all rancid, they need to be replaced, too.

Storage:

Store your dried herbs and spices in a dark, cool place. Many people store them near the stove where they are often exposed to heat, light and moisture.

When using herbs and spices, be sure to measure them before you get near a steaming pot. That can cause them to clump and you could ruin an entire jar of them.

Do It Yourself:

For those of you who feel inspired and like to make things, you will find Camina Gillotti's "Seasonal Spice Blends" on pages 87-88. You will also find some of my favorite herb and spice blend mixes. They are wonderful to use or make and give away as gifts.

I am sure that it would require an entire book to highlight all the beneficial herbs and spices (which is just about all of them) so I decided that I'd touch on those that I consider extremely beneficial and tasty for daily cooking. Using them daily is one of the keys to good health.

Nutrition Briefs:

Basil has been generally thought of as a culinary herb but it is loaded with Vitamin K, has antibacterial and anti-inflammatory effects, might help lower cholesterol, and is packed with potent antioxidants. When you eat pesto you get a great dose of basil. So when it's in season make your pesto and put it in your freezer for later in the year to perk up dishes. Or just add chopped basil to salads and soups.

Cayenne peppers, and other chilies, help stimulate blood flow which may speed up metabolism and help with weight management. In the 1400s, and likely earlier, chilies were the best available source of Vitamin C. They contain amazing amounts of vitamins and potent antioxidants. So, if you can stand the heat, add chilies to your food as powdered spice or whole chilies (or hot peppers), fresh or dried. Use small amounts in cooking as the heat often intensifies during the cooking process.

Cinnamon naturally sweetens food and appears to be important in blood sugar regulation which is good since cinnamon is often used in combination with sugar in sweet desserts. Sprinkling cinnamon on your oatmeal daily is a very good idea.

Ginger is useful for digestive disorders especially nausea. I find it useful to eat candied ginger to help with preventing car, and sea, sickness. It also tastes great. If you are not feeling well, add grated fresh ginger to hot water with lemon and make tea. It will likely perk you up.

Parsley adds freshness to many dishes, contains good amounts of Vitamin C and anti-oxidants. It is one of the most often used herbs. Don't forget to use it as a garnish often on your cooked dishes.

Turmeric is the main component in curry powder which is a mix of a variety of spices. This is why curry powders vary widely as each person can make their own blend. Curry powder does not have to be hot and spicy. Turmeric has the highest antioxidant activity of any of the spices and its active component, curcumin, has been shown to be highly anti-inflammatory. In some countries they grate fresh turmeric on the skin in areas that are inflamed. I recommend using turmeric often, as they do in India where the rates of dementia and other brain ailments are very low.

Herbs and Spices Flavor Profiles

Here is a short list of flavor profiles that might help you when you are trying to figure out how to season some of your dishes to make them taste a particular way. I have included a few items beyond herbs and spices to increase your flavor knowledge.

Chinese: black bean sauce, chilies, chili sauce with garlic, cilantro, garlic, ginger, hoisin sauce, dried shiitake or black mushrooms, plum sauce, sesame seeds, soy sauce or tamari, vinegar

Greek: bay leaves, cinnamon, dill, lemon, marjoram, nutmeg, oregano, pine nuts, rosemary

Italian: basil, garlic, dried mushrooms, oregano, parsley, rosemary, sundried and fresh tomatoes

Mexican: chilies (fresh, dried and smoked), chili powder, cilantro, cumin, garlic, onion, oregano, tomatillos, tomatoes and tomato sauce

Middle Eastern: allspice, cinnamon, cumin, garlic, lemon juice, parsley, pistachio nuts, sumac, tahini

Herbs and Spices Flavor Families

Here are the categories into which the herbs and spices fall. While I will only explore some of them, this is great information to know to aid in boosting flavors when cooking.

Sweet: allspice, anise, cardamom, cinnamon, cloves, nutmeg

Hot: chili peppers, garlic, onion

Spicy: cinnamon, ginger, pepper, star anise

Pungent: black pepper, celery seed, cilantro, cumin, curry powder, ginger

Herbal: basil, dill, marjoram, oregano, parsley, rosemary, sage, thyme

— Jill Nussinow

Garden Bruschetta

—CAROLYN SCOTT-HAMILTON—

This is a recipe to make in the peak of summer when all the ingredients are fresh and delicious.

Makes 4–6 appetizer servings

1 tablespoon olive oil

1 small red onion, finely chopped

1 eggplant, diced

2 cloves garlic, crushed

2 teaspoons soy sauce, tamari or *Bragg Liquid Aminos*

1 cup chopped artichoke (about the contents of 1 can)

3 large Roma tomatoes, diced

1 handful basil

1 teaspoon Dijon mustard

10 black olives, pitted and chopped

Salt and black pepper, to taste

Loaf of French bread (or crusty bread of choice), sliced and lightly grilled, for serving

Sauté the onion in a skillet with the oil (use vegetable broth instead of oil for a lower calorie dish)

Turn up the heat, add the eggplant and stir-fry until soft, approximately 10 minutes. Lower the heat, add the garlic, tamari, artichoke and tomatoes, followed by the basil, mustard, and olives. Gently sauté for a further 5 minutes.

Season and serve on grilled French bread or crusty bread slices.

Perfect Pesto Stuffed Mushrooms (raw)

—CHEF AJ—

When Rip Esselstyn came to my home for dinner the first time he ate the whole dozen by himself!

Serves 12

12 large Crimini mushrooms or Baby Bellas

1 cup pine nuts

2 cloves garlic

1 tablespoon yellow miso

1 cup fresh basil

Juice of one lemon, or to taste

Remove stems from mushrooms and set aside. Remove some of the center if necessary. Place the rest of the ingredients in a food processor fitted with the "S" blade and process until smooth. Fill the mushroom cups and dehydrate 2–4 hours until warm.

Chef's Note: If you don't have s dehydrator, bake in a 350°F oven for 45 minutes or until soft.

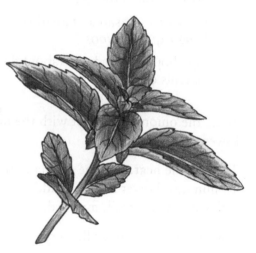

Stuffed Herb Pesto Holiday Appetizers

—KAREN RANZI—

This version of pesto is incredibly fresh and tasty.

Makes about 1 cup

⅓ cup pine nuts, soaked 20 minutes

½ cup parsley, chopped

½ cup basil, chopped

½ cup cilantro, chopped

1 tablespoon lemon juice

2 cloves fresh garlic, minced (optional)

1 tomato, chopped

Zucchini rounds

Bell pepper pieces

Mushroom caps

First grind the pine nuts in a food processor. Add the fresh herbs and process until finely chopped. Spread pesto on each mushroom, pepper or zucchini piece, and dehydrate at 105°F for 3–4 hours or until desired texture.

Pesto can be made in advance and marinate overnight in the refrigerator. For a final touch, a sliced olive can be added to the top of each dehydrated pesto appetizer before serving.

Carrots Stir-fried
with Mung Sprouts and Vegetables
—GITA PATEL—

Carrots contain vitamins A, C and K and the mineral potassium. Carrots and colored peppers contain the antioxidant beta-carotene. If you don't have the other vegetables you can stir-fry just the carrots with the sprouts, or carrots with cabbage but be sure to use all the spices which are full of antioxidants. This dish goes well with rice or beans.

Serves 6

1½ cups shredded green cabbage

1 cup grated carrots

½ cup sliced green onions

1 cup colored peppers, diced

2 cups packed mung bean sprouts

1–2 tablespoons canola oil

½ teaspoon black mustard seeds

Pinch of asafetida (hing), optional

2 tablespoons shredded, unsweetened coconut

⅛ teaspoon salt or to taste

⅓ teaspoon turmeric powder

¼ teaspoon cayenne pepper

½ cup cilantro with tender stems

1 tablespoon lemon juice

Assemble and prepare all ingredients.

Combine vegetables, sprouts, coconut, salt, turmeric and cayenne; set aside.

Heat mustard seeds in a 2-quart pan or skillet.

Before the seeds begin to pop, add oil, asafetida and vegetables with combined ingredients, stir well and cook for 5 minutes or to taste.

Add cilantro and lemon juice before serving.

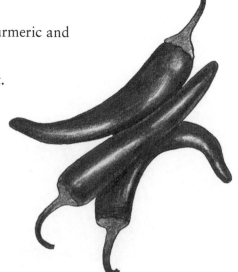

Cocoa-Spice Roasted Squash

—JILL NUSSINOW—

This sweet and spicy dish gets great balance from the addition of cocoa powder to the spice mix.

Serves 4

2–3 delicata squash or 2 acorn squash, to equal about 2 pounds

2 teaspoons canola or other neutral oil

2 tablespoons cocoa powder

2 teaspoons paprika plus more for garnish

½ teaspoon chili powder (not chili blend or hot chili powder but mild)

¼ teaspoon cumin powder

1 teaspoon *Sucanat* or organic brown sugar

Pinch of cayenne pepper

¼ teaspoon freshly ground black pepper

¼ teaspoon salt

Wash and cut squash into rings. Remove seeds and place rings in a 9-inch by 13-inch glass baking dish. If they don't fit well, use a second dish so that they all go into the oven at once.

Brush squash rings with the oil.

Combine the cocoa powder and remaining ingredients in a small bowl. Rub half the cocoa mixture onto the squash and turn squash over. Rub remaining mixture on squash.

Cover dish and bake for 20 minutes. Uncover dish and bake another 10–15 minutes until squash are easily pierced with a knife. Use a spatula to remove the squash rings to a platter.

Serve hot, dusted with paprika.

Cilantro Avocado Dressing

—JILL NUSSINOW—

This dressing is best when avocados are ripe and abundant. While this dressing works well on green salad, it also adds another dimension to tofu or tempeh and turns leftover grains or beans into a delicious salad.

Serves about ¾ cup

1 clove garlic

¼ cup packed cilantro

2 pitted Medjool, or other, dates

2 tablespoons lime juice, from 1 lime

1 medium avocado, in large pieces

¼ teaspoon salt, optional

Add garlic, cilantro and dates to a small food processor. Pulse until well chopped. Add the lime juice, avocado and salt. Process until almost smooth. Add a bit of water if the dressing needs thinning. Will keep for 3–4 days in the refrigerator.

Tomatillo Black Bean Salsa

—JILL NUSSINOW—

You can use any bean that you have on hand, or no bean at all and just use the vegetables. Get the best tomatillos that you can. Make it hot, or don't. It's up to you. I like to add toasted cumin for the best flavor.

Serves about 1½ cups

1 pound tomatillos, chopped, about two cups of chopped tomatillos

1 cup cooked black beans, rinsed and drained or freshly cooked

½ cup chopped onion

2–3 cloves garlic, minced

1 jalapeño, seeded and minced (optional)

1–2 teaspoons toasted cumin powder

½ cup cilantro, chopped

1 small lime, juiced

¼ cup chopped avocado (optional)

Salt and black pepper, to taste

In a medium bowl, combine all of the prepared ingredients except avocado. Stir that in carefully so that it remains intact. Taste and adjust the seasoning if necessary (more lime juice, salt and pepper, etc.).

Blueberry Gel

—FRAN COSTIGAN—

This soft and creamy dish has an especially beautiful color thanks to the blueberries, which are as healthful as they are delicious.

Serves 4–6

¼ cup (4 tablespoons) agar flakes

4 cups organic, no sugar added apple juice

1½ cups fresh blueberries, picked over, rinsed, and patted dry (or use frozen berries)

1 teaspoon ground cinnamon

2 tablespoons arrowroot

2 tablespoons filtered water at room temperature

Measure the agar into a medium saucepan. Pour in the juice, but do not stir or heat. Set aside for 10 minutes or longer to allow the agar to soften. This step will help the agar dissolve thoroughly and easily.

Bring the liquid to a boil over medium heat. Reduce the heat to low, and stir to release any bits of agar that may be stuck on the bottom of the saucepan. Cover and simmer for 7–10 minutes, stirring a few times. Uncover and check the juice in the saucepan, examining a large spoonful for specks of agar. If necessary, cover and simmer longer, until the agar has completely dissolved. Uncover, and add the cinnamon and blueberries. Simmer 1 minute if using fresh berries and 2–3 minutes if using frozen berries.

Combine the arrowroot with the water in a small bowl and stir with a fork to dissolve. Add the dissolved arrowroot to the simmering juice mixture, whisking constantly. Cook over medium heat only until the liquid boils. Immediately remove the saucepan from the heat. (If you cook or stir arrowroot-thickened mixtures after they have boiled, they are likely to become thin again.)

Pour into a bowl and cool for 15 minutes. Cover and refrigerate 30–40 minutes, or until set. Spoon the set gel into a food processor and pulse a few times until creamy. Pour into a serving dish or individual dishes. Store leftover gel in a covered container. It will keep for 2–3 days in the refrigerator.

Note: If you can only get agar agar powder, use 1 tablespoon (3 teaspoons) instead of the flakes but the flakes are preferred.

Variation — Blueberry Sauce: Purée a portion of the gel in a blender or food processor with enough additional juice to achieve the consistency you like.

Spiced Cauliflower

—GITA PATEL—

Cinnamon helps regulate blood sugar. Here it's combined with cauliflower which provides nutrient support for the body's detoxification system, its antioxidant system and its inflammatory and anti-inflammatory system, all closely connected with cancer development.

Serves 4

1 stick cinnamon

4 whole cloves

3 whole green cardamom

1 tablespoon canola oil

1 large tomato, diced

4 cups cauliflower florets in bite-sized pieces

1 teaspoon ground cumin

2 teaspoons ground coriander

1/8 teaspoon cayenne pepper, or to taste

1/4 teaspoon salt

3 tablespoons ground cashews

1/2 cup cilantro, chopped, for garnish

Assemble and prepare all ingredients. Heat a heavy-bottomed 2-quart pan with cinnamon stick, cloves and whole cardamom pods broken open slightly.

When the cloves begin to give out their aroma and darken add the oil and tomato, stir, and cook for 1–2 minutes.

Add cauliflower stir and cook covered till crisp tender. Add coriander and cumin powders, cayenne, turmeric, salt and cashews. Mix well and turn heat off.

Garnish with cilantro and serve.

Braised Cabbage with Cumin

—JILL NUSSINOW—

Cabbage is a nutrition powerhouse that's available all year. The cumin seeds might help make the cabbage more digestible and certainly add an intriguing flavor. This simple dish tastes better than it sounds.

1 minute high pressure; quick release

Serves 4

2 teaspoons canola, or other neutral, oil, optional

1 teaspoon cumin seeds

1 red or white onion, diced

6 cups finely chopped cabbage

3–4 tablespoons vegetable broth

Sprinkle of salt

Heat the oil in a pressure cooker over medium heat. Add the cumin seeds, onion and cabbage and sauté for 2–3 minutes. Add the broth and pressure cook for 1 minute. Quick-release the pressure. Sprinkle with salt to taste.

If you don't have a pressure cooker (quick, run out and get one), use ½ cup liquid and cook in a sauté pan for 5–7 minutes until cabbage is cooked through and you have the desired amount of liquid.

Ginger Lime Carrot Soup

—TESS CHALLIS—

This soup is pure, vibrant, delicious health in a bowl! If it were any healthier, it might be illegal in certain states. In fact, let's just keep this between you and me.

Serves 4

One medium sweet potato, baked until soft (1 cup sweet potato flesh)

3 medium-large carrots, peeled and chopped to equal 1½ cups

2 cups plus 1 additional cup plain, unsweetened non-dairy milk

2 tablespoons grated fresh ginger

1 tablespoon fresh lime juice

2 large cloves garlic, minced or pressed

1¼ teaspoons sea salt

¼ to ½ teaspoon ground cayenne (½ teaspoon will make it very spicy)

¼ cup chopped cilantro

Bake the sweet potato if you haven't already done so. Remove the skin and set aside.

In a medium pot, place the carrots in 2 cups of the non-dairy milk. Cover and bring to a boil over medium-high heat. Reduce heat to low and simmer, uncovered, until the carrots are tender. This should take about 20 minutes.

Place the sweet potato in a blender along with the carrots and milk. Add the additional 1 cup of milk and all of the remaining ingredients (except the cilantro).

Blend well, until very smooth. Serve immediately, topped with cilantro. Let the moaning begin!

Gingered Cucumber Salad

—JILL NUSSINOW—

This is an easy to make fat-free salad that is great for the late spring and all summer as it does not have to be refrigerated to taste good. Because I can get them, I usually use a combination of Armenian, regular and lemon cucumbers. Use what you can find, English cucumbers work well. Cucumbers are usually one of the first vegetables, after radishes, to show up at the spring farmers' markets.

Serves 4–6

½ red onion, sliced thinly

4–5 tablespoons of rice wine vinegar

3 medium or 6 small cucumbers, use some lemon cucumbers for color variety

2 teaspoons finely grated ginger

2–3 tablespoons toasted sesame seeds, for garnish

Combine onion and 2 tablespoons vinegar in small bowl. Let sit for about 10 minutes or more until the onion turns pink. Discard the vinegar.

Thinly slice cucumbers. Don't peel unless skin is bitter. Put into glass or ceramic bowl. Add soaked onion, remaining vinegar and ginger. Cover bowl. Stir at least once in 24 hours. Marinate at least 1 day. Add toasted sesame seeds, if you like.

Note: This low calorie dish will last up to four days in the refrigerator.

Ginger-Pineapple Pudding

—HEATHER NICHOLDS—

Who doesn't like a cool and refreshing pudding once in a while? This one actually aids your digestion, too.

Serves 4–6

2 cups non-dairy milk

1 cup pure pineapple juice

1-inch piece of fresh ginger, grated

2 tablespoons pure maple syrup, to taste

4 tablespoons arrowroot powder

1 tablespoon agar powder*

Mix all of the ingredients together in a small pot until thoroughly combined. For a milder ginger flavor, squeeze the juice from the grated ginger and leave the pulp out. If you really like ginger flavor, use all the pulp. You may not need any maple syrup with the sweetness of the pineapple juice, but it adds a nice flavor.

Put the pot on medium-high heat, stirring constantly until the mixture thickens. Don't let it get to a full boil, just a light simmer. Be sure to keep stirring as it thickens, and take the pot off the heat as soon as it gets to the consistency you like.

This is fantastic served with some pineapple chunks stirred in, and toasted coconut flakes sprinkled on top.

---

*Agar powder is different from agar flakes. If you use flakes you'll need much more than if you use powder.

Lime and Ginger Fruit Salad

—JILL NUSSINOW—

This is a simple way to jazz up already incredible summer fruit and make it work as a party dish.

Serves 4

4–6 peaches, nectarines, pluots or plums, or a combination, sliced
Juice of ½ to 1 lime
½ teaspoon grated ginger root

Agave, or maple, syrup, to taste
Handful of sliced strawberries or raspberries
Mint for garnish

Place sliced fruit in a bowl. Combine lime juice and ginger and pour over fruit. Mix gently but well. If fruit is really sweet, you do not need to add any sweetener. Let sit for at least 10 minutes and up to 30 minutes before serving. Garnish with berries, and mint, if desired.

Super Spring Salad
with Zesty Orange Dressing

—JILL NUSSINOW—

This salad has a combination of greens with a perky dressing. Citrus is in season this time of year, so you might as well take advantage of it.

Serves 4

4–6 cups salad greens (and reds, too)
1 cup bitter or other greens
1 orange, sectioned
¼ cup sliced red or green onion

DRESSING

½ cup freshly squeezed orange juice
1 teaspoon grated orange zest

¼ cup water
2 tablespoons mellow white miso
1 clove garlic, minced
½ teaspoon grated ginger
1–2 teaspoons agave syrup or other sweetener

Put greens in a bowl or on a plate or platter. Arrange orange on top.

Blend all dressing ingredients in the food processor (small) or blender until smooth. Pour over salad. Serve immediately.

Jill's Mustard Blend

—JILL NUSSINOW—

As you know mustard is part of the cruciferous vegetable family but the seeds are often used as a spice which is why this is included here.

Making mustard is quite easy. The quality depends on the quality of your ingredients. You can add any spices you like and use any type of vinegar or sweetener that you want. You can even add dried fruit, jalapeno peppers, horseradish, raspberries or other ingredients that you think would be tasty.

You can vary the mustard's consistency by grinding the seeds to a powder or leaving them whole or partially ground. Remember to let the flavor mellow for a couple of days or up to a week before tasting it to adjust any seasonings.

Because this mustard recipe doesn't use any eggs, it is less likely to break down or spoil. For the best results, store in the refrigerator.

Makes about 1½ cups

½ cup of combination light and dark mustard seeds

3 tablespoons dry mustard powder

½ cup water

⅓ cup balsamic vinegar

3 tablespoons rice wine vinegar

3 tablespoons maple syrup

½ teaspoon salt

1 clove garlic, minced

Combine mustard seed and mustard powder in a blender and blend until coarsely ground. Put into a small bowl and stir in water. Let sit at least 2 hours, stirring once or twice (if you have time or remember).

Put into blender with remaining ingredients and process until desired consistency. Put into a clean glass jar and let sit for 2–3 days before using.

If you find that the mixture is too liquid for your liking, place in the top of a double boiler and cook for 5–10 minutes to achieve the desired consistency.

This will keep indefinitely in the refrigerator and can be stored at room temperature in a cool, dark place.

Gutsy Greek Gigantes Beans
with Greens, Oregano and Mint

—ELLEN KANNER—

Beans, spinach, oregano, mint, lemon, garlic — these simple Mediterranean staples come together in a rustic dish that's as soulful and satifsying as it is nourishing. Beans offer fiber and protein, spinach has vitamins C, K, calcium, iron and more. Even oregano provides antibacterial and antioxidant properties as well anti-clotting Vitamin K.

Serves 6

2 tablespoons olive oil, plus another drizzle for serving, if desired

Pinch red pepper flakes

12 ounces dried gigantes beans or large lima beans, cooked, cooled and drained (about 4 cups of beans)

3 cloves garlic, minced

Grated zest of 1 lemon

2 tablespoons fresh lemon juice

2 tablespoons fresh oregano leaves, chopped (a few sprigs)

2 tablespoons fresh mint leaves, chopped (a few sprigs)

Sea salt and fresh ground pepper to taste

2½ ounces fresh spinach leaves (about 3 large handfuls)

Heat olive oil in a large skillet over medium-high heat. Add pepper flakes. When they start to sizzle, add the well-drained gigantes or limas. Spread beans out to prevent crowding.

Let beand cook for about 5 minutes, stirring occasionally to prevent sticking. When they start to brown on one side, flip them over and add the minced garlic and grated lemon zest. Reduce the heat to medium. Pour in the fresh lemon juice.

Continue cooking, stirring now and then, for another few minutes, until beans are lightly brown on both sides and are starting to develop a little bit of a crust. Add the chopped oregano and mint. Season generously with sea salt and fresh ground pepper.

Add the spinach leaves by the handful. Stir in gently and let the greens wilt — about 5 minutes. Gently toss again and taste for seasoning.

Serve with an extra thread of olive oil on top, if desired.

Herbed Tofu Dressing

—JILL NUSSINOW—

Tofu makes a great base for salad dressing as it has very little of its own flavor. Here it's blended with herbs which make it taste very fresh. This is great if you like creamy dressings. Add any other fresh herbs you like.

Makes slightly more than 1 cup

1 (12.3 ounce) box *Mori-Nu* firm or extra firm, lite or regular tofu

1 clove garlic, roughly chopped

3 tablespoons chopped herbs of any type, basil and parsley work well

3–4 tablespoons vegetable stock or water

1–2 tablespoons vinegar, any type will work

½ teaspoon salt

Combine all ingredients in a blender or food processor until smooth. Taste and add vinegar, garlic or salt to taste.

Herby Italian Dressing

—JILL NUSSINOW—

The artichoke hearts give this dressing some body. Only use frozen, bottled or canned in water, not the marinated ones.

Makes 1 cup

2 tablespoons vinegar

2 tablespoons onion, chopped

1 small clove garlic, cut in half

1 tablespoon apple juice concentrate, *Sucanat*, agave syrup or a few drops stevia

2 tablespoons chopped Italian parsley

¼ cup water

2 tablespoons basil

Pinch dried Italian seasoning

Fresh ground pepper, to taste

1 teaspoon reduced sodium tamari

½ cup artichoke hearts, frozen, thawed and cooked, or canned or bottled in water

Combine all ingredients in blender. Blend until smooth. Chill for at least 15 minutes before serving.

Parsley Pistachio Lime Pesto

—HEATHER NICHOLDS—

Parsley is loaded with nutrients — especially Vitamin K, folate, iron, Vitamin C and Vitamin A — so I use it when I can, especially to make a tasty recipe.

I used pistachios in the recipe, but you can easily substitute pumpkin seeds. Both pistachios and pumpkin seeds are high in iron, magnesium, manganese, potassium and phytosterols. Pistachios stand out for energy-supporting B vitamins, while pumpkin seeds are especially high in immune-boosting zinc.

I love to use this pesto spooned on top of a warm soup, as a sandwich spread or as the base for a yummy vegetable pizza.

Makes about 1 cup

1 cup fresh parsley

½ cup pistachios or pumpkin seeds

1 clove of garlic

1 teaspoon lime zest (optional)

2 tablespoons fresh lime juice

Pinch fine sea salt

1 tablespoon olive oil (optional)

1 tablespoon tahini or ¼ avocado (optional — for a creamy pesto)

Cut off any tough stems from the parsley, put all the ingredients in a food processor and purée until smooth. You'll need to scrape down the sides every so often to keep things combined.

Roasted Beet Hummus
with Thyme

—KAMI MCBRIDE—

I like to cook up a big batch of chickpeas and then store some in the freezer so I can whip up a batch of hummus any time. This humus is a crowd pleaser and the perfect dish to take to potlucks or holiday gatherings.

Serves 4–6

2½ cups cooked chickpeas

1½ cups roasted beets, chopped

1 cup roasted parsnips, chopped

2 cups soup stock (or water)

⅓ cup lime juice

½ cup tahini

2 tablespoons olive oil

1½ cups chopped parsley

1 cup chopped green onions

4 cloves garlic

1 teaspoon sea salt

1 tablespoon thyme

CHICKPEAS PREPARATION

5 cups chickpeas

9 cups water

2 2-inch pieces kombu seaweed

Soak chickpeas overnight in water. Strain water. Put strained chickpeas in a pot with 7 cups water and 2 two-inch pieces kombu.

Bring chickpeas to a boil, then cook on low heat until chick peas are soft but not mushy. Use some for this recipe and put the rest in a Mason jar and freeze for another recipe.

Prepare beets and parsnips. Chop beet and parsnips into 1-inch sized pieces. Cook in the oven at 350°F until beets and parsnips are soft.

Put all ingredients into food processor and blend until smooth and creamy.

Garnish with fresh thyme sprigs.

Mushroom Thyme Sauce

—MIYOKO SCHINNER—

This oil-free sauce is quick and easy, and yet elegant. Its richness and umami come from the mushroom stock and cashews, and its fragrance from thyme. Serve over tofu, tempeh, veggies, or a savory pastry concoction.

Makes about 1½ cups sauce

1 quart mushroom stock, either homemade or store-bought

2–3 tablespoons soy sauce or tamari

½ cup raw cashews

1 cups water

2 tablespoons chopped fresh thyme, or 2 teaspoons dried thyme

1–2 tablespoons cornstarch or arrowroot, dissolved in a little water

Place the stock and soy sauce in a 2-quart saucepan and heat. Combine the water and cashews in a blender and purée until smooth and creamy. Add the thyme to the stock mixture. Pour in the cashew mixture and simmer until slightly thickened. Mix in the cornstarch or arrowroot mixture to thicken more until a glaze consistency is reached.

Broccoli
with Turmeric, Ginger and Garlic

—JILL NUSSINOW—

I cooked at a garden called "Harvest for the Hungry" where they grow amazing organic produce that they give away to those who need it. I was given the most beautiful fresh broccoli heads to use and thought that they deserved special treatment that would enhance their flavor. This combo works well with most of the cruciferous vegetables. If you like a bit of heat, splash on some hot sauce.

1 minute high pressure; quick release
Serves 4

1 tablespoon oil (optional)

1 cup sliced onion, sliced from top to bottom

1 teaspoon minced fresh ginger

1 teaspoon grated fresh turmeric or ½ teaspoon dried powder

3 cloves garlic, minced

1 head broccoli, cut into florets, stem peeled and chopped

3 tablespoons broth

¼ teaspoon salt

Heat the oil and sauté the onion for a minute. Add the ginger, turmeric and garlic and sauté another minute. Add the broccoli, broth and salt. Lock on the lid and bring to high pressure. Set the timer and quick release the pressure after 1 minute.

Note: If you don't have a pressure cooker, make this in a sauté pan using ½ to ⅓ cup vegetable broth, as needed, simmering the mixture over medium heat until the broccoli is bright green and cooked to your liking.

Quick Lentil and Eggplant Curry

—JILL NUSSINOW—

The key to curry is the spices that you use. You can use a pre-made curry powder blend or you can make your own with turmeric, cumin, cardamom, coriander, cloves, chili powder, cinnamon or your favorite spices.

Serves 4

- 1 tablespoon canola or other vegetable oil
- 1 medium onion, diced
- 2 cloves garlic, minced
- 1–2 teaspoons grated ginger
- 1 cup mixed red and orange bell pepper, diced
- ½ cup red lentils
- 1–1½ cups vegetable stock

- 1 small eggplant, peeled and diced
- 3 small potatoes, cut into 1-inch pieces
- 1–2 tablespoons curry powder
- 1 small yellow squash
- 1 tomato, chopped
- ½ cup chopped apple or dried apricots
- Salt to taste

Put a pan over medium heat. When it is hot add the oil and then the onion. After 5 minutes add the garlic and ginger. Sauté for 3 minutes. Add the peppers, red lentils and 1 cup of the stock, the eggplant, potatoes and curry powder. Stir well.

Simmer for 15 minutes or until lentils, eggplant and potatoes are cooked through. Add more stock, if necessary. Stir in the yellow squash, tomato and chopped apple or apricots. Cook another 5 minutes until tomato is broken down. Add salt to taste. Garnish with cilantro or parsley.

Kale Apply Curry

—ELISA RODRIGUEZ—

This dish provides a hearty whole grain and legume combo with powerful anti-inflammatory properties from the garlic, ginger and turmeric. Use these natural seasonings to "clean house" in your spectacular cells. Enjoy a hint of sweetness from the granny Smith apple with plentiful greens peeking through. Top with freshly cut lime followed by freshly plucked herbs and your tastes will savor the spring season!

Serves 4–6

1 large yellow onion, finely chopped

3–4 garlic cloves, minced

1-inch ginger, minced

1 (15-ounce) can of organic chickpeas, rinsed well or 1½ cups cooked chickpeas

2 tablespoons curry powder (or 1 tablespoon cumin and 1 tablespoon of turmeric)

2–3 stalks of chopped celery

1–2 Granny Smith apples, chopped

4 cups of vegetable stock

A splash to ½ cup non-dairy milk

1 bunch finely chopped kale

1 handful fresh cilantro or other fresh herb

½ cup raisins (or other favorite dried fruit, apricots, dates) — optional

Freshly squeezed lime or lemon juice (not from concentrate)

A bed of cooked quinoa or brown rice

In a large pot, water sauté the chopped onion, garlic and ginger. Cook for a few minutes. Add the chickpeas and curry powder and continue to stir over medium heat.

After a few minutes of melding those flavors together, add the chopped celery, apples, vegetable stock and non-dairy milk.

Bring to a boil and reduce the heat. Add the kale, herbs and raisins. Cook, covered, over low to medium heat for 20–35 minutes until the mixture is cooked through but still bright green.

Serve over a bed of freshly cooked quinoa or brown rice, top with fresh herbs and a splash of fresh lemon or lime juice.

Seasonal Spice Blends

—CAMINA GILLOTTI—

Making your own spice blends means that you can add what you like and leave out what you don't.

Spices not only enhance the flavor of food but also help with digestibility. In Ayurvedic cooking, choosing spices according to each season can help to maintain balance and health. For example, it can be beneficial to choose more warming spices in the fall, pungent spices in the winter, bitter spices in the spring, and cooling spices in the summer. The following blends are designed to be specific for each season, but can be used with a variety of foods at any time of year. By using whole, fresh spices and herbs whenever possible, the most medicinal properties, flavors and aromas are extracted and infused into the food.

Once the blend is made (except the Summer Seasoning Blend), *transfer into an air tight container and store at a cool room temperature. Use your spice blend within the season to maintain potency and freshness. Each blend makes about ¼ cup.*

Summer Seasoning Blend

4 teaspoons fresh basil

4 teaspoons fresh mint

2 teaspoons fresh parsley

2 teaspoons fresh thyme

2 teaspoons fresh marjoram

1 teaspoon fresh lemon zest

Finely chop the fresh herbs and mix together. This blend is a good base for salad dressings with oil, salt, pepper, and vinegar; or sprinkled on top of grilled or steamed summer garden vegetables; and tossed into fruit salads. Once the herbs have been chopped, use immediately.

Fall Seasoning Blend

2 teaspoons whole fennel seeds
4 teaspoons whole coriander seeds
4 teaspoons whole cumin seeds
4 teaspoons powdered turmeric

1 teaspoon powdered ginger
2 teaspoons salt
½ teaspoon asafoetida (hing)

Lightly dry roast the fennel, coriander, and cumin seeds for two minutes. Grind the seeds with either a spice mill or electric grinder, and mix together with the other powered spices. Dry roasting and using whole seeds give a fuller taste, but you can also make this blend with powdered fennel, coriander, and cumin. Try these spices with bean and rice dishes, lentils, and cruciferous vegetables.

Winter Seasoning Blend

4 teaspoons cardamom pods
2 teaspoons whole cloves
1 teaspoon black peppercorns
5 sticks of cinnamon

2 teaspoons whole star anise
½ teaspoon salt
Sliced fresh ginger (optional)

To make a delicious spiced chai or add this blend to to apple cider, first boil 4 cups of water and add whole spices (except cardamom). Let simmer 15–20 minutes and keep the lid on the pot to contain the essential oils. Turn off the heat, add cardamom, and let sit for 10 minutes. Lastly, strain out all of the herbs For warm cereals and fruit compotes, blend together the powered form of each spice (for this recipe you will need 2 teaspoons of cinnamon). Enjoy sprinkled on top of oatmeal or even apple slices.

Spring Seasoning Blend

4 teaspoons whole coriander seeds
1 teaspoon celery seeds (ajwan)
1 teaspoon whole fenugreek seeds
1 teaspoon yellow mustard seeds

½ teaspoon ground ginger
½ teaspoon ground turmeric
½ teaspoon salt
pinch of cayenne or chili powder

Grind coriander seeds, celery seeds, fenugreek seeds, and mustard seeds with a spice mill or electric grinder. Mix together with powered herbs and use for cooking curries, dhals, dips, or sprinkle on top of salads or popcorn for a spicy snack.

All Purpose Salt-Free Spicy Mix

—JILL NUSSINOW—

This flavorful mix makes cutting down on salt easy. It doesn't take long before you adjust to being salt-free.

Makes about ¼ cup

1½ teaspoons each dried parsley, sage and thyme

1 teaspoon each dried rosemary, paprika, oregano and celery seed

1 teaspoon each garlic powder and onion powder

1 teaspoon ground black pepper

3 tablespoons nutritional yeast flakes

Combine all ingredients in a blender and process until powdered so that flavors combine. Use a funnel and transfer to a nice bottle or spoon into a tin. Use daily to season your food.

Cocoa Spice Powder

—JILL NUSSINOW—

This is a good as a rub on vegetables, tempeh or tofu.

Makes about ¼ cup

1 teaspoon ground black pepper

1 teaspoon ground coriander

1 tablespoon ground cinnamon

1 teaspoon ground cumin

1 tablespoon cocoa powder (unsweetened)

1–2 teaspoons chipotle chili powder or 2 teaspoons paprika

¼ teaspoon salt

Combine all ingredients in a small bowl and transfer to a bottle. Use or give as a gift.

Herb and Chile Rub

—JILL NUSSINOW—

This was inspired by a rub made by Chef Jeffrey Beeson at The Point Hilton Resort at Tapatio Cliffs *in Phoenix, Arizona. He grows all the herbs and spices in his garden. "We go to the store and still come out with a terrific product that can be rubbed onto meat, fish, poultry or even tofu before grilling. It also makes a good daily spice blend."*

You can also do this with paprika instead of chilies, and omit the cayenne, for a milder blend.

Makes ¼ cup

1–2 dried chilies (depending on size), cut into pieces — use ancho or pasilla or any that you like (or you can use a good chili powder, not spice)

1½ teaspoons cumin seeds, toasted

1 teaspoons coriander seed

1 tablespoon garlic granules or 2 teaspoons powder

¼ teaspoon cayenne pepper

1 teaspoon oregano

1½ teaspoons onion powder

1½ teaspoons thyme

1 teaspoon rosemary (optional)

1 teaspoon sage (optional)

1½ teaspoons black pepper (optional)

2–3 teaspoons *Sucanat* or brown sugar

Combine all ingredients except sugar in a spice grinder or blender. Blend until smooth. Pour into a bowl, stir in the sugar and put into a container.

Spiced Nuts

—JILL NUSSINOW—

These are quite easy to make, they taste great and are easily packaged to look nice in cellophane bags with ribbon or rafia. You can use whatever spices you like such as curry or cinnamon, cardamom and cloves. Almost anything works.

Makes 2 cups

- 2 cups shelled nuts, can use almonds, walnuts, pecans or other of your choice
- 2 teaspoons canola oil
- 2 teaspoons *Bragg Liquid Aminos*
- 1 teaspoon cumin powder
- 1 teaspoon chili powder
- ¼ to ½ teaspoon chipotle powder or cayenne pepper
- 2–3 teaspoons *Sucanat* or organic sugar

Heat a non-stick pan over medium heat. Add the nuts and let toast for 3 minutes. Meanwhile, combine the canola oil, *Bragg Liquid Aminos* and spices in a bowl.

After the nuts have toasted, pour them into the bowl and stir to coat with the oil-herb mixture. Return to the pan and toast for another 2 minutes stirring occasionally. Lower the heat a bit and sprinkle the sugar over the nuts. Cook 1 more minute, shaking the pan every once in a while. Turn off the heat and let the nuts sit about another minute.

Put on a baking sheet to cool. They are now ready to package.

CHAMPS

Alliums Included

Garlic

Green Onions

Leeks

Onions

Shallots

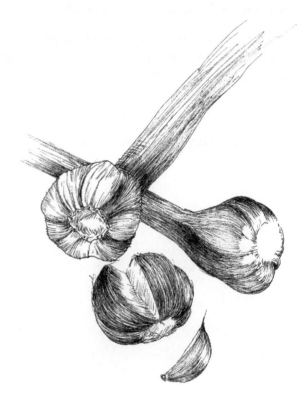

CHAPTER 3

Alliums

THE ALLIUM FAMILY which includes chives, garlic, leeks, onions and shallots is what I consider the backbone of cooking. They are used throughout the world except in certain cultures in Indian, Japan and China where some monks and sects consider them too stimulating, which makes me know that they are tasty. I could probably start each recipe by sautéing, or dry sautéing, onions and garlic and my husband will want to know what I am cooking. The aroma is tantalizing and brings back memories of my mother and grandmother's cooking.

Generally leeks and onions are interchangeable in recipes although leeks have a milder flavor, despite being a tougher vegetable. Shallots are used in recipes much less often because they are harder to grow and store which makes them more expensive to purchase. They can stand in for leeks or onions even though they generally have a milder flavor, especially when cooked. Shallots are a wonderful addition to salad dressing based on vinegar. Chives are most often used for garnishes, especially if they have their beautiful purple flowers intact which are completely edible.

The alliums are freshest when they are harvested, which is generally spring, except for garlic. Many people do not realize that garlic is a fresh crop. Garlic is usually planted in October or November and harvested in June. Then it is cured, usually by hanging the long stems, until July or August to let the bulbs dry. Green garlic is harvested in the early to late spring and you can eat the entire stalk from unformed cloves, at the bulb, end and all the way up the stem, if it's not too woody, which it should not be. The flavor is milder than cured garlic. If you are unusually lucky, you might be able to purchase garlic "scapes" which are the curly tops of hard neck garlic which are harvested to add value to the farmers' garlic crop. They can be added to soups, grilled outdoors or used any way that you like them.

There are many types of garlic which all have different flavors and amounts of heat. If you are lucky you will have someone near you who grows specialty garlic. If not, you can buy garlic online and plant your own.

The nutritional benefits of all alliums has been known for centuries which is probably how we've come to know that eating garlic will keep vampires away. My theory is that eating garlic often keeps "germy" people away which keeps you healthier, especially in the winter when germs tend to linger. Actually, garlic is extremely anti-bacterial due to the compounds that it contains.

To activate the beneficial allyl sulfide compounds in garlic, the garlic needs to be cut or crushed, even before cooking, and then it needs to sit for at least 10 minutes to activate the compounds. Eating it raw is beneficial but cooking it is fine as long as it is quickly cooked. Some studies have shown that prolonged cooking, for more than 20 minutes, significantly decreases garlic's effectiveness to fight bacteria.

In addition to garlic's beneficial antimicrobial compounds, it might also be effective for lowering cholesterol and helping with blood pressure regulation.

Green onions, which are called scallions in certain parts of the United States and the world, are the best source of the antioxidant flavonols, a compound similar to that found in green tea. Green onions have a beneficial effect on cardiovascular disease risk. They are easy to use and eat, raw or cooked and make a great addition to salads as they tend to be much milder than onions or shallots. I usually use the entire stalk, both green and white, if it is tender enough.

Leeks are often used in French cooking wherein they mostly stick to using the white part of the vegetable. Just so you know, the entire stalk is edible so where color doesn't matter so much, feel free to add the darker green part of the leek. Note though that it is often more fibrous than the white part.

Onions and shallots are a rich source of quercetin which is an antioxidant, with antimicrobial and antibacterial properties that likely help stimulate your immune system. They are good for you whether eaten raw or cooked, and if you tolerate them both ways, eat them as such. Shallots contain much more quercetin than onions but we eat far fewer of them for the reasons stated above.

All allium peels and trimmings, unlike the cruciferous vegetables, add incredible flavor to stock and are often the basis for making good stock. Although the vegetables are cooked, I bet that good nutrition passes into the liquid although I have no scientific proof of this (so please forgive me for being presumptuous here but if wonderful aroma is any indication of nutrition, then I could be correct).

All the vegetables in the allium family contain sulfur, as do they cruciferous vegetables which make them strongly flavored and aromatic, as well as making them good for you. Additionally they are sources of prebiotics which help regulate good bacteria in your gastrointestinal tract. Eating alliums regularly might help lower the incidence of colon cancer, as well as all the other stated nutrition benefits listed above.

What I like best of all, of course, is how they make your food taste great easily. So get cooking with some alliums today.

Allium Broth

—JILL NUSSINOW—

This broth can be used for daily cooking instead of using water, in which case I'd freeze it in ice cube trays which will give you a tablespoon or two at a time. Or you can use it as a soup base for soup such as Potato Leek or any garlic based soup.

Makes 7–8 cups

2 tablespoons minced garlic
   (1 large or 2 small heads)

1 medium onion, chopped

1 leek, cleaned well and sliced

8 cups water

1 sprig fresh sage or ½ teaspoon
   dried sage

3 sprigs Italian parsley

1 sprig fresh thyme

Salt and ground black pepper, to
   taste

Dry sauté the garlic, onion and leek in a large pot over medium heat. Cook until the onion is transparent, adding small amounts of water, if necessary to prevent sticking. Add the 8 cups of water and herbs and bring the mixture to a boil.

Reduce the heat to a simmer. Simmer covered for 15–30 minutes. Strain. Season with salt and pepper.

This will keep in the refrigerator for 1 week and it freezes well.

Note: If you use a pressure cooker, you can make this recipe by adding the water and bringing to high pressure for 5 minutes. Then let the pressure come down naturally. Carefully remove the lid and strain.

Creamy Caesar Salad Dressing

—JILL NUSSINOW—

This makes your Caesar salad sing. If you want to make it with less fat you can substitute one half a carton of Mori-Nu Lite silken tofu for the almonds and water. This will last for up to a week in the refrigerator but it's doubtful that you will have it hanging around that long.

Makes 1 cup

¼ cup almond meal or ⅓ cup soaked almonds, drained and ¼ cup water

4 cloves garlic

3 tablespoons Dijon mustard

¼ cup nutritional yeast flakes

1 tablespoon tamari or soy sauce

1 tablespoon vegetarian Worcestershire sauce, optional

3 tablespoons lemon juice

2 tablespoons water or more depending upon consistency you want

Place the almonds or almond meal in a small food processor with the garlic and pulse until the garlic is minced. Add the water, mustard, yeast flakes, tamari, Worcestershire and lemon juice and process until smooth. in the blender and blend until smooth, adding additional water if necessary.

Drizzle as much as you need over chilled, washed and torn Romaine lettuce that has been topped with croutons.

Garlic, Greens, and Tofu
with a Twist

—JILL NUSSINOW—

What's fresh at the market this week? Toss it in. I hope that you learn to love this dish as much as I do. It's my go-to meal for breakfast, lunch or dinner, at least once a week, yet it rarely tastes the same way twice. The sweetness of the preserves offsets the slight bitterness of the greens. You can use any type that catches your eye.

Serves 4

1 tablespoon oil, optional

1 medium onion, diced

2–3 small potatoes such as fingerlings or purple type, cut into 1-inch pieces

2 cloves garlic, minced

1 stalk green garlic, minced

1 piece ginger root, minced or grated

½ pound firm tofu, cubed

1–2 tablespoons tamari, *Bragg Liquid Aminos* or soy sauce

¼ cup or more broth or water

3–4 cups, or more, of assorted greens, sliced thin (kale, collards, turnip, mustard or your favorite)

2 tablespoons preserves such as apricot or orange marmalade

1 teaspoon lemon zest and 2 tablespoon fresh squeezed lemon juice

A pinch of chili paste, hot sauce or chili flakes

Salt and pepper, to taste

Cilantro, for garnish

Heat a sauté pan over medium heat. Add the oil, if using, and let heat. (If omitting oil, use dry sauté method.) Add the onion and sauté for about a minute, adding a tablespoon of water or broth as soon as the onion begins to stick. Add the potatoes, garlic, ginger, tofu and tamari and sauté for another 10 minutes, adding the rest of the broth, as needed.

When the potatoes are almost cooked through, add the greens and cook until the greens turn bright green, in 3–5 minutes.

Stir in the preserves and lemon juice. Add chili, salt and pepper, to taste. Garnish with chopped cilantro (optional)

Did You Say Green Onions?

Perhaps where you live green onions are called "scallions." They are a member of the allium family, which also includes bulb onions, leeks, garlic, shallots and chives. When the shoots are young and tender they often look similar.

One time I went to New Orleans for a food technology conference — to find a convention hall filled with artificial flavors, colors, starches, gums, additives and very little that resembled food. I yearned for something fresh and couldn't wait to get home to real food.

I was eager to arrive at the San Francisco airport and be back on familiar turf. My now husband Rick was in the car waiting for me at the curb when I walked outside the terminal.

I threw my bags in the back seat and sat down in the front next to Rick. I noticed that he didn't smell like his usual self. He reeked of garlic. Rick likes garlic and will eat it but avoids eating it raw or in copious amounts. Since I arrived in the morning I was surprised at the stench. As politely as I could, I asked, "What did you have for dinner last night?"

"I made a salad and put in that bunch of green onions that you had in the frig," he replied.

I laughed, "That explains it. You cut up an entire bunch of green garlic and ate it on your salad last night. You really smell like garlic." He was completely unaware. I often tell my students this story so that they have some warning.

So, be sure that you can tell the difference between green onions and green garlic. Obviously it was easy for Rick to confuse the two since he doesn't buy the food or make the salad. Usually if you crush a leaf and sniff you will know. Also garlic and leeks have flat leaves and spring and green onions are round with a hole. If you're still not sure, taste it. But don't worry if you confuse them because someone will let you know, hopefully politely.

—Jill Nussinow

Garlic Herb Aioli

—JILL NUSSINOW—

My friend recently told me that she likes buying pre-made vegan garlic aioli. I shudder to think of how much fat it contains. This one has plenty of flavor and not much fat. Use it as a dip for vegetables, as a spread on sandwiches or as a dressing for potatoes or vegetables.

Makes about 1 cup

- 1 (12.3 ounce) box of *Mori-Nu Lite* silken tofu
- 4 cloves garlic, minced fine
- 2 tablespoons mellow whire miso
- ¼ cup fresh lemon juice
- 1 tablespoon capers
- 2 tablespoons fresh Italian parsley
- 2 teaspoons Dijon mustard
- 2 teaspoons nutritional yeast
- 2 pinches cayenne pepper
- ½ teaspoon sea salt, optional
- 2 tablespoons water

Place all in a blender and purée. Stores up to a week. Has the consistency of mayonnaise. Add more water if it seems too thick.

Garlic Sesame Broccoli Salad

—MORGAN ECCLESTON—

I can usually find toasted sesame seeds in Asian markets or well stocked grocery stores. If you can't find them you can always toast your own at home. Cook in a dry pan while stirring constantly over high heat for 4–5 minutes or until toasty.

6 Servings

- 1 pound of broccoli, cut into bite sized florets
- 5 cloves garlic, minced
- 1 teaspoon toasted sesame oil
- 1 tablespoon rice vinegar
- 2 tablespoons toasted sesame seeds
- 1 tablespoon low sodium tamari

Bring a large pot of water to a boil. Add the broccoli florets. Cook for 1 minute. Drain the broccoli and plunge into a bowl of ice water to stop the cooking. Let cool and drain.

Whisk together the remaining ingredients. Toss with the broccoli. You can serve immediately or refrigerate and serve chilled.

Garlicky Lemon Spinach Salad
with Sunflower Seeds, Olives and Sprouted Beans

—JILL NUSSINOW—

Spinach is so delicious, especially combined with the flavors of lemon, olives and garlic. Eating the raw garlic keeps you healthy in the winter. The sprouted beans turn this into a complete meal.

Serves 4

6 cups small spinach leaves

¼ cup toasted sunflower seeds

2 cups mixed salad sprouts, including sunflower

2 cloves garlic, crushed

3–4 tablespoons regular or Meyer lemon juice

1 teaspoon Dijon mustard

2 tablespoons flax or flax blend oil, optional

½ to 1 teaspoon *Sucanat* or sugar

3 tablespoons Kalamata olives, chopped

Salt and pepper, to taste

Put the spinach in a large bowl. In a separate bowl, blend the garlic, lemon juice, mustard and oil. Whisk together. Pour over the salad. Add salt and pepper. Top with the seeds, sprouts and olives. Serve immediately.

Note: If you use regular lemon juice, you may want to add a pinch of sugar to balance out the flavors.

Tofu and Snow Pea Stir Fry Salad

—CAROLYN SCOTT-HAMILTON—

These simple ingredients combine to make a tasty salad that is perfect for lunch or dinner.

Serves 4

- 1 pound tofu, pressed, drained and cubed
- 14 ounces vegan chicken broth (store bought or made from vegan chicken bouillon)
- 3 tablespoons rice vinegar
- 3 tablespoons reduced-sodium soy sauce or wheat free tamari
- 3 teaspoons toasted sesame oil, divided

- 2 tablespoons tahini or cashew butter
- 1 tablespoon minced fresh ginger
- 2 cloves garlic, minced
- 1 pound snow peas, trimmed and thinly slivered lengthwise
- 2 tablespoons chopped cashews

Place tofu in a medium skillet or saucepan and add broth; bring to a boil. Cover, reduce heat to low, and simmer gently until cooked through, 10–12 minutes.

Transfer the tofu to a plate or bowl to cool. Cool and refrigerate the broth, reserving it for another use.

Meanwhile, whisk vinegar, soy sauce, 2 teaspoons sesame oil and tahini (or cashew butter) in a large bowl until smooth. Set aside.

Heat the remaining 1 teaspoon oil in a large nonstick skillet over medium heat. Add ginger and garlic and cook, stirring, until fragrant, about 1 minute. Stir in slivered peas and cook, stirring, until bright green, 3–4 minutes. Transfer to the bowl with the dressing.

Add the tofu to the bowl with the peas; toss to combine. Serve sprinkled with cashews.

White Bean Garlic Soup

—JENN LYNSKEY—

This light soup is the perfect start to a meal of tapas or if you're feeling under the weather. Although the ingredients are simple, use the freshest garlic and a rich homemade stock or a good quality un-chicken type broth at about 1½ strength.

Serves 2

8 cloves garlic

1½ cups rich vegetable stock divided

1 cup cooked white beans

Salt to taste

In a blender, blend together 1 cup of vegetable stock and white beans until smooth.

Peel garlic and slice in half lengthwise, then slice thinly.

In a medium sauce pan over medium heat, add remaining ½ cup stock and garlic slices. Heat for about 5–7 minutes or until the broth has evaporated and the garlic is soft and mellow. Then sauté another minute. Add the bean mixture and cook until heated.

Serve immediately in a shallow bowl.

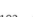

Lemon Scented Spinach Spread

—JILL NUSSINOW—

This is a tasty way to get people to eat more vegetables. It is far healthier than the spinach dip that many have gotten used to that is based on mayonnaise (or even veganaise). You can use this to make wrap sandwiches as well as putting it in a traditional "bread bowl."

Makes 1½ cups

- 1 (10-ounce) package frozen chopped spinach, thawed, drained and squeezed dry
- ½ cup chopped green onions
- ½ (12.3-ounce) package *Mori-Nu Lite* silken tofu
- ¼ cup fresh lemon juice, to taste
- 1 teaspoon lemon zest (be sure to zest before juicing)
- 2 teaspoons Dijon mustard
- 1–2 teaspoons *Sucanat* or sugar, to taste (optional)
- Salt and pepper, to taste
- Lemon zest and lemon slices for garnish

Combine the spinach and green onions in the food processor and pulse. Add the tofu, lemon juice and zest, and mustard. Process until smooth. Add salt, pepper, lemon juice and *Sucanat*, to taste.

Serve immediately after making it or make a day ahead and serve chilled. If you make it ahead be sure to taste before serving as sometimes the flavors get muted. Garnish with twisted lemon slices and lemon zest strips.

Baby Leeks á la Nicoise

—JILL NUSSINOW—

Leeks are often overlooked in this country. They have a terrific flavor, especially when roasted. If you really like them, as I do, you may need to increase the number of leeks per serving. Roasting without oil is difficult as the oil is what helps the vegetables get a bit caramelized. You can do it with just a tablespoon or two of broth or wine and they will taste good, but just won't brown much.

Serves 4–6

8–12 baby leeks about ¼ inch in diameter, washed well, top few inches of green removed

1 tablespoon olive oil, optional

2 teaspoons fresh thyme or ¾ teaspoon dried thyme

Salt and pepper, to taste

2 tablespoons red wine vinegar

2 cloves garlic, minced

1 cup peeled, chopped, fresh or canned tomatoes

Pinch of cayenne pepper

Fresh thyme and chopped Italian parsley, for garnish

Preheat oven to 350°F.

Put the leeks on a parchment lined baking sheet and drizzle the olive oil over them, if using. Sprinkle the thyme on top of leeks and move them around to be sure that they are coated with oil. Bake in the oven for 20 minutes until they are getting browned.

While the leeks are roasting, combine the red wine vinegar, garlic, tomatoes and cayenne. After 20 minutes of roasting, add the liquid mixture to the leeks and bake another 10 minutes.

Serve hot, sprinkled with thyme and parsley.

Leek and Butternut Squash Soup

—LAURA THEODORE—

The delicate flavor of leeks enhances fall favorites like butternut squash and parsnips, making this hearty soup a real crowd-pleaser. Purple cabbage provides a deep and inviting color and the brown rice thickens the soup, while adding substance. This tummy warming fare is the perfect potage to serve during cold weather months and beyond.

Makes 6 servings

2½ cups sliced leeks, white and light green parts (see note)

2 cups peeled, seeded and cubed butternut squash

2 cups sliced carrots

2 cups sliced purple cabbage

1½ cups sliced parsnips

1 cup chopped green beans

1 clove garlic, minced

¾ cups whole grape tomatoes

½ cup uncooked short grain brown rice

1 teaspoon Italian seasoning

1 teaspoon brown sugar or maple sugar (optional)

¼ teaspoon sea salt

32 ounces vegetable broth

Filtered or spring water, as needed

Put the leeks, squash, carrots, cabbage, parsnips, green beans, garlic, tomatoes, rice, Italian seasoning, optional sugar, and salt into a large soup pot. Add the vegetable broth and enough water to cover the vegetables.

Cover and bring to a boil over medium heat. Decrease the heat to medium-low and simmer the soup for 1 hour or until the vegetables and rice are soft and the soup has thickened.

Serve in pretty soup bowls with crusty whole grain bread on the side.

Note: Leeks must be cleaned thoroughly to remove the fine sand and dirt often embedded between the layers. Here's a quick and easy way to do the job: Split the leeks lengthwise. Put them in a large bowl filled with cold water and soak briefly to loosen any debris. Then rinse the leeks thoroughly under cold water, parting the layers slightly so the debris rinses away. Put the leeks in a clean bowl of cold water and swish to remove any remaining sand or dirt.

Leek and Potato Soup

—JAIME KARPOVICH—

It seems as if leeks and potatoes were made for each other.

Serves 4–6

3 large leeks

2 tablespoons water, plus more
  if needed

2 cloves garlic, minced

3–4 white or yellow potatoes

8 cups vegetable broth

½ cup unsweetened non-dairy milk

Slice the leeks in half lengthwise, rinsing grit out of the leaves. Slice the leeks into small half-moons. Add with the water to a soup pot over medium-high heat. Add more water, as needed, until leeks are soft, about 5–7 minutes. Add garlic and sauté one minute.

Chop potatoes into bite-sized pieces, leaving the skins on if they are organic. Add potatoes and broth to leek mixture and bring to a boil, then simmer until potatoes are soft.

To make it even creamier, blend one third of the soup in a blender and add it back to the soup pot.

Baked Stuffed Onions

—JILL NUSSINOW—

Cooking and opening the onions takes a bit of work but the ingredient list is easy to put together. They make quite an impression when served. Adding a salad makes this a complete meal.

Serves 4

- 4 large onions
- 2 cups cooked quinoa or bulgur
- 8 ounces fresh spinach, steamed, squeezed dry, and chopped
- 2 tablespoons chopped Kalamata olives
- 2 tablespoons finely chopped walnuts, plus more for a topping
- 3 tablespoons fresh chopped Italian parsley
- 2 tablespoons nutritional yeast
- 1/8 teaspoon freshly ground nutmeg
- 1/4 teaspoon freshly ground pepper
- 1–2 tablespoons lemon juice

Preheat the oven to 375°F. Peel the onions, leaving the root end intact.

Set up a steamer basket above at least 1 cup of water in a medium pot. Put the onions on the rack with the root side up. Steam for 15–20 minutes, until the onions are tender enough to be pierced by a skewer but still feel a bit crunchy.

Remove the onions with a slotted spoon, and set the root end down on a flat baking dish. Let them stand until they are cool enough to handle.

To hollow the onions, slice off the top fourth of each onion. Using a small pointed knife, make several cuts into the center of the onion, going about two-thirds of the way down to the bottom and cutting to within 3 or 4 of the outermost layers. When the center of the onion has been well scored and the interior layers feel loose, hollow out the center with a teaspoon or a melon baller, leaving a wall of at least 3 layers, about 1/4 inch thick. Coarsely chop what you have removed from the onion center and cut off a small part of the root end so that the onion stands but still holds together.

Combine all the remaining ingredients in a large bowl to form the stuffing.

Arrange the scooped out onions in the baking dish. Pile in the stuffing, mounding it in the center of each onion. Top each onion with a sprinkling of walnuts.

Bake until lightly browned on top, about 20–25 minutes. Let stand for a few minutes before serving.

Curried White and Sweet Potato Pancakes
with Fresh Fruit Chutney

—JILL NUSSINOW—

This variation on traditional potato pancakes makes them even tastier. Grating the potatoes in the food processor makes the recipe quicker. Onions are always essential to making tasty potato pancakes. You can bake these pancakes in a 375°F. oven for a total of 20 minutes on parchment or silpat lined baking sheet instead of frying them.

Makes 20–30 small pancakes

1½ pounds large potatoes, like russets or Yukon gold, grated

1½ pounds sweet potatoes or garnet yams, grated

1 large onion, grated

1 tablespoon egg replacer mixed with ¼ cup water

¼ cup all purpose, whole wheat pastry flour or gluten-free flour blend

1 teaspoon baking powder

½ teaspoon salt

1 tablespoon curry powder

2 tablespoons canola oil, optional (see note about baking)

Mix the potato, sweet potato and onion together well in a large bowl. Squeeze out any excess liquid and drain. Add the egg replacer mixture, flour, baking powder, salt and curry powder and mix well.

Add 1 tablespoon of oil to a large non-stick skillet over medium heat. Place ¼ cup batter for each pancake into the skillet. Cover with a lid until the bottoms are golden brown, about 5 minutes. Flip to the other side and cook until golden brown. Serve hot with chutney.

If the pancakes are done and there are still more to cook, which there will be, then put them on a baking sheet in a 300°F oven to keep warm.

Fresh Fruit Chutney
with Mustard Seeds and Cilantro

—JILL NUSSINOW—

This fruit chutney can spice up many dishes in the winter. Here it is a perfect accompaniment to the mixed potato pancakes.

Makes 1 cup

Juice of 1 lime

1 apple, unpeeled and diced

¼ cup minced red onion

1 tablespoon maple syrup

1 tablespoon raspberry vinegar

1 tablespoon black mustard seeds, toasted

2 tablespoons chopped fresh cilantro

Squeeze the lime juice over the diced apple. Combine with the rest of the ingredients and let sit for at least 15 minutes before serving.

Note: If you want this chutney to be hot, mince a half a jalapeno or hotter chili and add it to the mixture.

Fat-Free "Forks Over Knives"-Style Onion Mushroom Gravy

—LANI MUELRATH—

Recently inspired to make gravy that is easy to put together, not full of fat, or out of a packet, I came up with this little gem. Keep in mind I do not like to spend much time in kitchen prep. But I do love to eat healthy, and eat well. That's why I'm working on cultivating some good kitchen attitude.

And with fall a quick turn of the calendar page away, what better to create than a healthy, savory gravy to go with all those colorful starchy vegetables? I call it "Forks Over Knives" mushroom gravy as it covers all the bases: Plant based, low fat, no animal products. I just jazzed it up a bit by calling it "F.O.K." gravy instead of "plant-based, vegan, low-fat, no-animal-products, mushroom gravy." Does that work for you? OK, so it breaks my usual recipe rule of no more than five ingredients. This one's worth it.

A Word about the Mushrooms

You could also switch out fresh mushrooms for the dried, but something about the dried blend is particularly savory. Also, if it is too dense in mushrooms for you, just use fewer next time. Serve over potatoes, sweet potatoes, riced potatoes, whole grains, vegetable loaf, vegetables... somebody stop me! Take a batch to the Thanksgiving table to share this year. After all, the other one on the table (warning, graphic in nature) is just blood and fat. Sorry kids. It's true. And F.O.K. Mushroom Gravy will leave you satisfied and feeling light without a monster calorie load.

Serves

- ½ sweet onion, finely chopped
- 2 cups dried mushroom blend, soaked
- 5 cloves minced or pressed garlic
- 2 cups water (I used the water from the soaked mushrooms as part of this; you could also use veggie broth.)
- 1 tablespoon vegetarian bouillon concentrate (exclude if using veggie broth)
- 1 teaspoon *Bragg Liquid Aminos* organic sprinkle herbs and spices seasoning
- 1 tablespoon nutritional yeast
- 1 tablespoon cooking wine (optional)
- ¼ cup non-dairy milk
- 2 tablespoons flour
- Fresh ground pepper, optional

Put the dried mushrooms (I used *Shiitake-ya* gourmet blend from *Costco*) in a container and cover with hot water. Let it sit at least an hour. I just let it sit all day. Drain just before using.

Steam-fry chopped onions and garlic veggie broth until golden. Add the mushrooms, chopped* if you like, and cook a few more minutes.

Add 2 cups water, taking whatever came off the mushroom soak and adding either plain water or vegetable broth, nutritional yeast, herbs, and cooking wine. If using vegetable broth, you can eliminate the bouillon and vice versa.

Stir the flour and rice, oat, or soymilk to a smooth paste, then add to the pan with the rest of the ingredients and keep stirring over low heat as it thickens.

Season with freshly ground pepper to serve, if desired.

---

* With the dried mushrooms, it is easy to break them up into bits before soaking, sparing you the chopping later.

Go-To Winter Medley

—ELISA RODRIGUEZ—

This winter medley has become one of my favorite go-to staples in the colder months of the year. It includes an ample blend of robust winter squash, wholesome quinoa and nutrient rich greens with seasonal colors, tastes and textures for an attractive, nutritious and delicious dish. It is free of dairy, gluten/wheat, corn, soy and nuts.

Serves 4–6

- 1 pound butternut squash, cubed and cut
- 1 large red onion, cubed
- 1 dash toasted sesame oil
- Black pepper, to taste
- 1 head dark leafy greens such as kale, collards or mustard
- 4 cups water

- 2 cups quinoa
- 1 no salt added vegetable bouillon cube from Rapunzel or homemade vegetable broth
- Raw, unsalted pumpkin seeds, as desired
- Dried cranberries, as desired
- Fresh parsley, to garnish

Preheat oven to 350°F.

Spread cubed butternut and onion on a large pan, and sprinkle with black pepper as desired. Drizzle a little bit of toasted sesame oil, for seasoning, and mix well with clean hands to evenly disperse the ingredients. Cover with foil. Add to the oven for 30–45 minutes.

Meanwhile, bring the 4 cups of water to a boil on your stovetop at medium heat. Add the vegetable bouillon (or you can use homemade veg broth here.) Allow the bouillon to dissolve prior to adding the 2 cups of quinoa. Allow the quinoa to simmer and expand on low heat.

Next, wash and prepare the head of greens. To water-sauté, add ¼ cup of water to a large pan on medium heat. Add the prepared greens, cover and allow to soften and wilt.

Once the quinoa pilaf has cooked for roughly 20 minutes, it can be dished up for serving. Top the quinoa with greens, followed by the butternut medley. Dress with pumpkin seeds, cranberries (for color and sweetness) and fresh parsley.

Roasted Stuffed Onions
with Carrot-Potato Purée

—LINDA LONG—

My father, in our diner, always advised using tons of onions as they cook down and give great flavor while supporting the other flavors. In this recipe the onion is the star, not a supporting player. Any large sweet onions will work!

Serves 6

6 large onions, unpeeled (about 8 ounces each)

2 tablespoons oil of choice for rubbing onions

2 medium carrots, peeled, roughly sliced into 1-inch pieces (about 10 ounces)

1 teaspoon salt

2 medium red potatoes, peeled, roughly cut into 1-inch pieces (about 14 ounces)

¼ cup non-dairy milk of choice, sweetened or unsweetened

Salt to taste

¼ teaspoon white or black pepper to taste

Preheat oven to 450°F.

Preparing the onions: Without peeling the paper-like outside skins cut a thin slice from the bottom root end of 6 onions that will allow them to set upright, and a larger slice from the top of each onion. Carefully rub the oil around the onions in preparation for baking. Place on a baking sheet and bake until soft, about an hour or slightly more. Once baked, use a turner underneath and tongs for sturdiness when removing to plates.

Preparing the purée: Place carrots and potatoes in a saucepan with enough water to cover and add the salt. Boil until tender, about 25 minutes. Carrots should be very soft. Drain.

Put into the bowl of a stand mixer or in a mixing bowl and use an electric hand mixer. Note that a hand masher can also be used but the purée might be less creamy. Start to gently beat the mixture until just mashed. Add some of the milk and beat on medium. Add more milk if the mixture is too stiff. The texture should be like fluffy mashed potatoes but still holding a shape. Note that some potatoes absorb milk more than others and thus need more or less. Taste for any need for more salt, and add pepper. Beat just enough to blend in any added salt and pepper.

Completing the dish: Remove onions and cool slightly. Remove skins and scoop out the center with a knife and teaspoon in such a way that the outside circumference remains strong. Save removed onion for a sandwich or to complement another vegetable dish. Fill the cavity and pile high above the onion with 1/3 cup of the mixture. If desired, place stuffed onions under the broiler to reheat and brown the top slightly. Serve with a serrated dinner knife for easier cutting. Use as a side dish or along with any grains, beans, or lentils to make it a main entrée.

Thai Bangkok Noodles

—JILL NUSSINOW—

This is an easy to prepare noodle dish with Thai flavors. You can omit the curry powder and use a teaspoon or two of Thai red, green or yellow curry instead but leave out the hot chile unless you are a "hot head." Shallots and green onions are often used in Thai cooking.

Serves 4

¼ cup vegetable broth

½ cup light coconut milk or coconut water

2 tablespoons *Bragg Liquid Aminos*, tamari or soy sauce

1 tablespoon curry powder, or to taste

½ cup sliced shallots

¼ cup chopped green onions

¼ teaspoon freshly ground black pepper

2 teaspoons vegetable oil, optional

2 teaspoons minced garlic

1 tablespoon chopped fresh galangal or ginger root

1 small hot fresh chile, minced

4 ounces firm tofu, cut into ½-inch cubes

1¼ cups mung bean sprouts

3 cups baby spinach

6 ounces rice vermicelli or other rice noodles, soaked in warm water for 20 minutes and drained

Lime wedges and/or chopped cilantro

Mix the broth, coconut milk, *Bragg Liquid Aminos*, curry powder, shallots, green onions and pepper together in a small bowl. Set aside.

In a large wok or skillet, heat the oil, if using, (if not using, dry sauté or add a bit of broth) over medium-high heat. Add the garlic, galangal, and chile. Stir-fry for 15 seconds. Add the tofu and stir-fry for 1 minute. Add the coconut milk, or water, mixture and bring to a simmer. Add half the mung bean sprouts, all the spinach and the noodles and stir-fry for about 30 seconds until the spinach starts to wilt.

Remove from the pan and put on a platter. Sprinkle with the remaining mung bean sprouts and a bit of lime juice. Garnish with lime wedges or cilantro.

C H A M P S

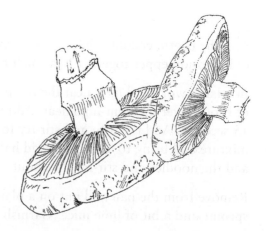

Mushrooms Included

Black Truffle

Crimini

Maitake

Oyster

Portabello

Shiitake

Trumpet

White

CHAPTER 4

Mushrooms: Fungi Fun

I HAVE ALWAYS LIKED mushrooms so eating them comes naturally to me. I asked a former student who was from Japan which mushrooms they eat in Japan for health and nutrition. She told me that there is "no difference." That is not the case here in the United States although mushrooms are tasty and texturally pleasing so they are often used in cooking.

More than ten years ago I became a mushroom hunter. I joined my local mycological association *(Sonoma County Mycological Association)* and I have never looked back. I have looked down, though, hundreds of times searching for signs of edible fungi.

As interesting as it is, my husband doesn't eat mushrooms. Some people call this a flaw but I love it. When I hunt, or just cook, them, there are more mushrooms for me.

Luckily we don't have to forage for mushrooms when we want to eat them. We can go no further than our local supermarket or natural foods store. I happen to live near a company that is one of the mushroom growing pioneers. *Gourmet Mushrooms* sells under the *Mycopia* label. They grow organic, "wild" cultivated mushrooms which include alba clamshell, brown clamshell, Trumpet Royale, maitake and more.

They don't grow any magic mushrooms, yet I believe that all mushrooms are magical, and not in a mind-altering, although perhaps palate-altering, way. How they grow and what they do for us and the planet sets them apart from other plant foods. In fact, they are not vegetables, they are fungi.

Well-known mycologist Paul Stamets says that we are more closely aligned with mushrooms than with plants, and that without fungi we would be buried in dead matter from our forests. So we need mushrooms.

When I began my mushroom research, the information that I gathered pointed to their amazing health benefits. I didn't yet understand the role that they play in human health and probably have for thousands of years, before people could put names to the special components in mushrooms.

Briefly, what makes mushrooms special is that they contain *chitin,* which is an indigestible component found in the exoskeletons of crustaceans and some insects.

The chitin helps move cholesterol out of our bodies. Mushrooms are also a source of a specific carbohydrate called *beta-glucans* which helps regulate blood sugar and spurs your immune system to do its best work.

All mushrooms are good for you, even some that cannot be eaten directly such as reishi and turkey tail which must be turned into tea, cooked into soup or consumed as tincture or capsules. Many others, even the common white button mushroom, have beneficial qualities. It turns out that mushrooms can concentrate Vitamin D from the sun. They also contain B vitamins and various minerals but most importantly for me, they add amazing texture and wonderful flavor to plant-based cooking.

Mushrooms have the fifth taste which is referred to as *umami,* a Japanese word for an indescribable flavor that is not sweet, salty, sour or bitter. One of the best sources of umami is shiitake mushrooms. Interestingly shiitake mushrooms also have potent anti-cancer properties. So, good taste and good health are rolled into one mushroom.

Studies have shown that consuming one-half ounce of dried blue oyster mushrooms daily for three months can lower your cholesterol by thirty percent which is as much or more than statin drugs but without side effects.

All over the world people are studying mushrooms for their role in health maintenance, disease prevention and as possible cures for a variety of ailments. Mushrooms have antibacterial, antiviral effect and provide a host of antioxidants which help scavenge free radicals in your body.

"The most fascinating aspect of medicinal mushrooms is enhancing the function and activity of the body's immune system." —Andrew Weil, M.D.

As you will see from the breadth of recipes, mushrooms are a wonderful addition to soups, stews, stir-fries, side dishes, veggie burgers and more. Mushrooms should always be thoroughly cooked as they contain a mycotoxin that is deactivated through cooking. There is a thought that since many of the components in mushrooms are water-soluble that it's best if you consume any mushroom cooking liquid.

Mushrooms are incredibly versatile and can be steamed, baked, roasted, grilled, sautéed, breaded and cooked in any way that you can think of. Their flavors are versatile, too, and they pair well with many herbs and spices used throughout the world. They are a mostly universal food, and can be found growing on every continent.

Many people are confused about how to store mushrooms. They are unfortunately usually sold in plastic bags or wrapped in plastic which is something very foreign to nature and the world in which fungi reside. They need air circulation. The best way to store mushrooms is in paper bags. They need to be used within three or four days so that they are in the best possible condition. If your mushrooms feel slimy, they are usually past the point of edibility.

People often want to know about washing mushrooms. Do not wash before storing them. Clean immediately before eating them. If they have dirt on them, you can use a brush or you can wash them but don't leave them soaking as they are what is known as hydrophilic (water loving) and will soak up water. A quick dunk or rinse is what commercially produced mushrooms need. Wild mushrooms are a different story, and one that I will not address here.

Mushrooms are low in calories and contain a lot of fiber so they fill you up. You can eat them daily or cook a lot at once and freeze them to eat later. You will be amazed at what mushrooms can do for you. Although, if you are like my confirmed "mushroom hating" husband you can always take mushroom supplements. However you get them, I consider them essential for great health.

A Brief Mushroom Primer:

Edible mushrooms: The recommendation is to eat three ounces fresh, cooked or 1/3 ounce dried at least three times a week. You will often need to rehydrate dried mushrooms. Be sure to use the strained, clean soaking liquid, which has lots of flavor in your cooking or just drink it.

Shiitake (*Lentinus Edodes*)**:** They have an earthy flavor and "meaty" texture when cooked. Remove woody stems and save for soup stock. Use in stir-fries, vegetable sautés, veggie burgers and loaves, stuff them or sauté them by themselves.

Oyster Mushroom (*Pluerotus Ostreatus*)**:** Many types of oysters are available and their colors can be quite spectacular, especially the pink and yellow ones. They all taste a bit different and are milder than shiitakes which makes them more adaptable to a variety of recipes. You can roast them on a parchment-lined baking sheet at 500°F until done. Or sauté and turn into mushroom tacos with corn and jalapenos and salsa.

Maitake, "hen of the woods" or "dancing mushroom" *(Grifola frondosa):* They may be good for inhibiting tumor growth and to lower blood pressure and cholesterol. They are delicious but expensive. Wonderful roasted or sautéed with garlic, ginger and tamari.

Mushrooms are low in calories and fat and do not contain cholesterol. They have more protein than most vegetables, have many minerals and are a good source of B vitamins. They contain considerable fiber so they fill you up without filling you out. Eating too many at once may give you an upset stomach.

Medicinal Mushrooms:

The very short list which I would be remiss if I did not include here:

Reishi or Ling Zhi *(Ganoderma lucidum):* "The most broad spectrum healer of all medicinal mushrooms," according to Paul Stamets of FungiPerfecti/Host Defenes. It is good for respiratory conditions: allergies, asthma and bronchitis. Strictly medicinal, it is hard, woody and bitter. Consume as tea, tincture or extract.

Cordyceps or caterpillar fungus *(Cordyceps sinensis):* Woody and tough, consume as tincture, tablets or capsules for overall health benefits.

Turkey Tail *(Trametes versicolor):* Grows abundantly in my part of the world and is highly medicinal. Can be made into tea or tincture, and can also be added to soup stock. They are a general health tonic for the immune system.

To Recap:

One of the unique compounds in mushrooms is *beta glucans,* which is a mega-sugar molecule that is also called a *polysaccharide.* Unlike refined sugar, these are beneficial sugars that help kick the immune system cells into action. This might explain the beneficial effects of shiitake mushrooms in cancer and HIV/AIDS treatment. For more information check out the book *Sugars That Heal* by Emil I. Mondoa, M.D.

Truffled Celeriac Soup

—LYDIA GROSSOV—

Celeriac is a gnarly-looking, knotted root vegetable (also known as celery root) derived from wild celery, which has a small, edible root and has been used in Europe since ancient times. But don't judge a book by its cover. Its delicate flavor of celery and parsley with a slight nuttiness — pairs wonderfully with black truffles — and silky smooth texture will delight your tastebuds. This soup is a great starter for a special occasion dinner or to treat yourself, just because.

Serves 4-6

5 small or 3 medium celeriac, peeled and cubed

1 small onion, diced

1 clove of garlic, minced

1 teaspoon extra virgin olive oil or 1 tablespoon water

¼ teaspoon nutmeg, freshly grated

3 cups of water

1½ ounces black truffle

Salt and pepper to taste

Black truffle oil (optional) and chives for garnish

Place the cubed celeriac in a medium sauce pan with water and boil until cubes are fork tender. Drain and set aside.

In a separate sauce pan, sauté the diced onion in olive oil, or in water for oil-free, until it begins to turn translucent. Add the minced garlic and continue to sauté until the edges turn golden.

Add the cooked celeriac, sautéed onion and garlic mix, whole black truffle, salt and pepper to taste, nutmeg and 3 cups of water in a food processor or high-speed blender cup. Blend until smooth and all ingredients are evenly incorporated. A high speed blender, such as a Vitamix, will make the mixture silkier and fluffier.

Plate the soup in your favorite bowl and garnish with black truffle oil (optional) and sprinkle with finely chopped chives.

Coconut-Chickpea Crepes
with Smoky Herbed Mushrooms

—ERIN WYSOCARSKI—

Packed with succulent mushrooms kissed with a hit of smoked paprika, these crepes make the perfect brunch or light dinner item.

Serves 4

FILLING

½ tablespoon olive oil

1 large shallot, cut in half, then thinly sliced

10 ounces mushrooms, thinly sliced

2–3 garlic cloves, halved and thinly sliced

½ teaspoon dried thyme

½ teaspoon smoked paprika

2–3 tablespoons coconut milk (skim the heavy part off the top of the can)

1 teaspoon coconut, or other,vinegar

Salt and pepper, to taste

CREPES

½ cup coconut milk

¾ cup sparkling water

½ cup chickpea flour

1 tablespoon tapioca flour

1 tablespoon nutritional yeast (optional)

A few dashes of salt

Olive oil, for sautéing

Chopped fresh parsley, for serving

To make the filling, heat the olive oil in a medium-sized sauté pan over medium-low heat. Place the shallots into the pan and sauté for about 3 minutes, stirring occasionally. Add in the mushrooms, then place a lid over the top. Increase the heat to medium and allow the mushrooms to sweat for 4–5 minutes. Remove the lid and slightly lower the heat to allow some of the moisture to evaporate, about 4–5 minutes more. Add in the garlic and sauté for an additional 2 minutes.

Add in the thyme and paprika. Stir well. Scoop off 2 or 3 tablespoons of the coconut cream from the top of the can. Reserve the rest of the canned coconut milk for the crepes. Add it to the pan and allow it to melt. Stir to combine, then add ½ teaspoon of coconut vinegar to the pan. Taste and add another ½ teaspoon, if desired. Season with salt and pepper to taste. Keep it over the lowest heat setting possible while you make your crepes.

To make the crepes, pour the remaining coconut milk into a bowl. Stir it until the thin and thick parts are thoroughly combined. Measure ½ cup and add it to another bowl, then add in ¾ cup of seltzer water. Whisk vigorously, then add in the chickpea and tapioca flours, nutritional yeast and salt. Whisk again.

Heat a clean non-stick circular pan over medium heat for 5 minutes. Spray with a little cooking spray or oil, then quickly pour a thin layer of the batter into the middle. Pick up the hot pan immediately and tilt the pan around so it is evenly covered with batter. Return the pan to the heat and allow it to cook until the edges are slightly golden brown, about 3 minutes. Carefully flip it over with a spatula, then cook for only 1–2 minutes more. This should make about 4 medium-sized crepes.

Spoon some of the mushroom filling into each of the crepes. Sprinkle with a bit of fresh parsley and serve immediately.

Lentil, Mushroom and Walnut Paté

—JILL NUSSINOW—

This makes a great holiday, or other special occasion, appetizer. It can be frozen if there is any leftover.

Serves 8–10 as an appetizer

1 cup dried green lentils

½ ounce dried wild mushrooms

2 medium leeks, white part only, chopped

½ pound crimini mushrooms, thinly sliced

2 large garlic cloves, minced

1 clove garlic, crushed

½ cup finely chopped toasted walnuts plus ¼ cup toasted halves for topping

1 tablespoon chopped fresh thyme or 2 tablespoons dried thyme

4 tablespoons quick-cooking or baby oats or oat flour

Salt and freshly ground pepper

¼ teaspoon paprika

2 tablespoons balsamic vinegar

4 tablespoons chopped Italian parsley

Pick over the lentils and put them in a pot. Cover with water and let them cook until they are soft, 35–45 minutes. (Or pressure cook for 6 minutes with a natural release.) Drain, reserving liquid, and set aside.

Pour boiling water over the dried wild mushrooms and let them soak for 15–30 minutes.

Heat the medium skillet. Add the leeks and dry sauté for 2–3 minutes. Squeeze the water out of the wild mushrooms (saving the water) and add the rehydrated mushrooms to the pan along with the crimini mushrooms, minced garlic and ½ cup walnuts. Cook over medium heat until the mushrooms release their liquid, about 10–13 minutes. Add the thyme and oats and cook for 4–5 minutes longer.

Purée the mushroom mixture in the food processor with the lentils and vinegar, adding ¼ teaspoon freshly ground pepper and ¼ teaspoon paprika. If the mixture seems too thick, add some lentil cooking liquid or mushroom soaking liquid. Taste and add salt, if necessary.

Line a 3–4 cup terrine or narrow 10-inch by 4-inch bread pan with parchment or wax paper.

Sprinkle the parsley and ¼ cup walnuts over the paper and add the lentil-mushroom mixture. Cover and refrigerate for at least 30 minutes until cooled down.

When ready to serve, unmold the paté by pulling at the paper lining to ease the paté from the sides of the pan. Set a platter over the paté and then invert. Ease the pan off the paté, then peel off the paper. Surround the paté with sprigs of parsley and cherry tomatoes, if in season.

Quick-Stuffed Crimini Mushrooms

—LAURA THEODORE—

These quick to prepare, but totally tasty stuffed mushrooms make the perfect side dish, starter course or appetizer for any festive meal. A pop of fresh basil compliments the rustic combination of chopped walnuts and whole grain bread cubes, while the garlic adds a punch of classic flavor.

Serves 4

- 8 ounces crimini mushrooms, cleaned and stemmed
- 1 large slice whole grain bread, diced
- 2 cloves garlic, minced
- 1 tablespoon fresh chopped basil, or 1 teaspoon dried basil
- 2 teaspoons finely chopped walnuts
- 1/8 teaspoon sea salt
- 1 tablespoon vegetable broth, plus more as needed

Preheat the oven to 350°F. Line a large, rimmed baking sheet with unbleached parchment paper. Place the bread, garlic, basil, walnuts and sea salt in a medium bowl. Stir to combine. Add the vegetable broth and stir gently to combine. If the stuffing seems dry, add more vegetable broth one teaspoon at a time until the mixture is moist, but not soupy.

Spoon a generous spoonful of stuffing into each mushroom cap and press it firmly into the cap. Put the mushrooms on the prepared baking sheet.

Cover and bake for 40 minutes. Uncover and bake 10 minutes more, or until the stuffing is crisp and golden.

Rich Mushroom Gravy

—JILL NUSSINOW—

This is great served over mashed potatoes. You can also serve this alongside stuffing at the holidays, or any day that you want to feel like a holiday.

Makes 3 cups

6 ounces crimini mushrooms, thinly sliced

3/4 cup spelt, whole wheat, brown rice or unbleached flour

1/2 teaspoon thyme

1/2 teaspoon black pepper

3 cups water

1/4 cup reduced sodium tamari

1–2 tablespoons raw tahini

2 teaspoons lemon juice

2–3 tablespoons nutritional yeast

Heat a saucepan over medium heat. Add the mushrooms and dry sauté for 5 minutes, until they start to brown and release a bit of liquid. Remove the mushrooms and set aside. Add the flour, thyme and pepper to the pan and stir constantly until the flour is toasted to a golden to medium brown. Gradually add water with a whisk to remove any lumps. When blended, add the mushrooms and the last 4 ingredients and mix well. Adjust the seasonings as needed. You can add a little bit of sugar or maple syrup for balance. Serve hot.

Variation: Soak 1/2 ounce dried mushrooms (such as porcini or shiitake) in 1 cup warm or hot water for 30 minutes. Use part of this soaking water (the part without dirt and debris) as the liquid for the gravy. Finely chop the drained, soaked mushrooms and add to gravy mixture before adding the last 3 ingredients.

Rosemary Mushrooms and Kale

—CATHY FISHER—

This one-pot recipe is very quick and easy to make, using just kale, mushrooms, yams, garlic and rosemary — yum! For this dish, I use curly kale because of its hearty texture and delicious peppery-ness.

Serves 4

1 cup water

2 large yams or sweet potatoes, skin on, cut into ½-inch slices

2 cloves garlic cut in half

2 bunches curly kale, roughly chopped, stem ends trimmed

12 large crimini mushrooms or 8 baby bellas (small portabellas)

4 sprigs fresh rosemary

Place 1 cup water in a soup pot with the yam slices and garlic and bring to a boil.

Place the kale on top followed by the mushrooms. Lay the sprigs of rosemary on top and cover. Decrease heat to medium-low and steam for 10–15 minutes, or until the yams are easily pierced with a knife. Serve immediately.

Dry Sautéing

Some authors of fat-free recipes suggest adding some type of liquid to pan "sauté" the initial ingredients, which for me often includes onions and garlic. If you use that method what you end up with are steamed or boiled vegetables instead being sautéed.

My technique requires that you have a heavy-bottomed pan such as stainless steel or a safe nonstick coating (but not Teflon). The pan manufacturers recommend that you cook on heat no higher than medium as the higher heat tends to burn the pan's nonstick coating. This is why I start with a dry pan over medium heat.

I call this technique dry sautéing. Put the pan over medium heat for a few minutes. Add the ingredients in the order listed and for the recommended cooking times. The key to preventing burnt food is to stir occasionally and look at the ingredients to be sure nothing is sticking or burning. If that starts happening, add water, broth, juice or wine, a tablespoon at a time so you can easily scrape off the stuck-on food particles. Do not add so much liquid that the ingredients get soggy, or you will not be sautéing. You will just be drowning your food.

I have found that dry sautéing is the best oil-free method for extracting the most flavor from food. This was confirmed when I saw Chad Sarno, who I think is one of the best plant-based chefs around, do a cooking demonstration using the dry-sauté method. It is one of the easiest ways I know for eliminating a tablespoon of fat and more than 100 calories from your diet.

— Jill Nussinow

Veggie Mushroom Burgers

—JILL NUSSINOW—

I used to make this burger using bread crumbs to hold it together but I no longer keep bread around and it's better for you to use more whole grains. So this has some ground chia or flax seeds as a binder. You can add any seasonings you like to this burger but I prefer to let the umami of the mushrooms and sundried tomatoes shine through. I cannot say that they will be wonderful on the grill but if you really like them, put some in your freezer to eat as a part of a quick meal.

Makes 6 burgers

Vegetable cooking spray or spray oil, optional

8 ounces crimini, shiitake or portabella mushrooms, chopped

½ onion, chopped to equal about 1 cup

3 cloves garlic

1 small carrot, cut in pieces

5 sundried tomatoes, rehydrated in ¼ cup boiling water, chopped fine, reserve water

1½ cups cooked brown rice, quinoa or bulgur

¾ cup cooked, cubed potatoes

¼ cup cashews

½ cup rolled oats, kamut, quinoa or other flakes

1 tablespoon lite tamari, optional

¼ teaspoon black pepper

2 tablespoons ground flax or chia seeds

Preheat oven to 375°F. Line a baking sheet with parchment. Spray with vegetable spray, if you like.

Combine mushrooms, onion, garlic and carrots in the food processor. Whir until the mushrooms are well chopped and the carrots are in small pieces. (Do not wash the processor yet.)

Spray a pan with cooking spray, if you want, or dry sauté, and add the mushroom mixture. Cook for about 5 minutes over medium heat until the onions are soft and the mushrooms have released some liquid. Transfer to a large bowl and set aside to cool.

Put the rice, sundried tomatoes, cashews and potatoes in food processor and process until the cashews are in small pieces — about 3–5 pulses. Add the seasoning, tamari and pepper. Add the mushroom mixture and process briefly with another 3 pulses.

If it seems too dry, add 2–3 tablespoons of the tomato-soaking liquid.

Transfer this mixture to the bowl that you have previously used and add the oats or other flakes, tamari, pepper and ground seeds. Stir a few times to combine.

Let the mixture sit for 5 minutes to firm up. Using wet hands, form into 6 patties about 3-inches in diameter and ½-inch thick.

Put the burgers on the prepared pan and bake for 12 minutes, then turn them. Bake for another 10 minutes or until crispy and brown. Let stand for a few minutes and then eat.

Note: You can pan-fry these in a nonstick pan if you don't want to use the oven. I prefer using the oven as I like them cooked all at once.

Wild Mushroom and Farro Stew

—JILL NUSSINOW—

Farro tastes nutty and has a firm texture. (To make this gluten-free use oat groats instead.) Combined with mushrooms of various types, it is hearty comfort food at its best.

Serves 4–6

1 tablespoon oil, optional

1 medium onion, diced

3 cloves garlic, minced

3 cups sliced crimini or white mushrooms

1 cup sliced shiitake mushrooms

¼ cup dried porcini or other wild mushrooms

1½ cups farro, semiperlato (which means semi-pearled)

4–6 cups vegetable stock

1 bay leaf

3 sprigs fresh thyme

Salt and freshly ground black pepper, to taste

Chopped Italian parsley, for garnish

Soy Parmesan, optional

Heat the oil in a medium saucepan over medium heat. Add the onion and sauté for 3 minutes. Add the garlic and mushrooms and sauté another 7 minutes. Add the farro, 4 cups of stock, the bay leaf and thyme sprigs. Bring to a boil and then reduce the heat to a simmer. Cover and let cook for 30 minutes and check the liquid level. If it seems too dry, add another cup of stock. When the farro is firm but cooked through, about 45 minutes, and the mixture is slightly runny it is done.

Remove the bay leaf and thyme stems. Stir in the salt and pepper. Serve garnished with parsley. Pass cheese on the side, if you like.

Pasta with Creamy Cashew Maitake Mushroom Sauce

—JENN LYNSKEY—

I originally made this with fresh maitake mushrooms that I got from the farmers' market, but it works just as well with dried maitake mushrooms. I found the dried mushrooms at an Asian market which were much less expensive than a health food store and they also came with the stem attached. If you don't plan ahead to presoak the cashews, soak in hot water for 10 minutes while you're preparing the other ingredients and they'll blend more easily.

Serves 4–6

1 cup dried maitake mushrooms

1 cup hot water

1 tablespoon soy sauce or tamari

½ cup raw cashews (preferably presoaked for 4 hours and drained)

1 cup water

1 small sweet onion roughly chopped

2 garlic cloves roughly chopped

4 fresh sage leaves roughly chopped (or 1 teaspoon dried)

1 pound whole wheat, or other, pasta cooked according to package directions

In a small bowl, add boiling water and soy sauce to the dried mushrooms and let sit for 10 minutes.

In a blender, mix soaked drained cashews with water, onion, garlic, and sage. Blend until smooth. Add mushrooms with soaking liquid and blend briefly on low to combine, but not long enough completely obliterate the mushrooms.

Pour the sauce into a large sauté pan to heat. You can add extra water if the sauce gets too thick. Add more soy sauce or salt to taste.

When pasta is cooked, add to the pan and toss to coat.

Serve immediately with fresh chopped sage for garnish.

Roasted Maitake

—JILL NUSSINOW—

This is such as simple dish to make. It doesn't take long to cook. Even though maitake tend to be pricier mushrooms, I think that their taste and superior nutritional qualities make them worth buying, cooking and eating. They also look like beautiful flowers.

Serves 4

8 ounces fresh maitake mushrooms, cut or pulled apart in 2-inch long pieces

2 tablespoons tamari

2 teaspoons toasted sesame oil or 1 tablespoon balsamic vinegar, for oil free

Freshly ground black pepper, to taste

Preheat oven to 400°F. Line a baking sheet with parchment paper.

Combine the tamari and oil or balsamic in a large bowl. Add the mushroom pieces and toss to coat. Place them, with plenty of room around them, on the baking sheet. Bake for 10 minutes. Remove from the oven and turn them over.

Bake another 5 minutes or until the mushrooms get crispy.

Note: You may also do this with thinly sliced Trumpet Royale mushrooms which are a type of oyster mushroom.

Oyster Mushroom, Asparagus and Tofu Stir Fry

—JILL NUSSINOW—

Get the freshest asparagus as you can since it is the star in this dish. If asparagus is out of season, use beautiful broccoli or green beans.

Serves 4–6

½ pound of tofu, cut into cubes

2 tablespoons tamari or soy sauce

1 tablespoon canola oil, optional

2 medium shallots, chopped fine

2 teaspoons finely minced ginger

½ pound of oyster mushrooms, cut in half or more depending on their size

1 pound of asparagus

½ teaspoon salt

¼ cup vegetable broth

½ teaspoon arrowroot or cornstarch

Finely ground black pepper, to taste

teaspoon lemon zest

Lemon juice, to taste

Marinate the tofu in the tamari while you prepare the other ingredients.

Break off the tough ends of the asparagus and cut the asparagus on the diagonal into 1-inch pieces, except for the tips, which you will leave whole.

In a small bowl, combine the broth, cornstarch, pepper and lemon zest.

Heat the oil over medium high heat in a large skillet or wok. Add the shallots and ginger and sauté for a minute, stirring often. Add the mushrooms and sauté for 5 minutes until they are starting to get limp but are not yet cooked through. Add the tofu, any unabsorbed tamari and the asparagus. Sauté for 3–4 minutes, stirring occasionally.

When the mushrooms have released their liquid and the asparagus is bright green and almost cooked through stir the broth mixture and pour into the pan. Stir well to coat all the ingredients. Taste. Add lemon juice, salt or pepper, if necessary.

Grilled Mushroom and Spring Onion Salad
with Miso Tahini Dressing

—JILL NUSSINOW—

Mushrooms, especially portabello and shiitake, and tamari have a flavor called umami which is indescribably delicious. Portabello are large crimini mushrooms with less liquid. Grilled spring onions are sweet. The dressing is rich and salty.

Serves 3-4

1 tablespoon tamari

1 teaspoon toasted sesame oil

1 teaspoon grated ginger

½ pound portabello mushrooms, sliced if large

1 medium spring onion, sliced

2 teaspoons mellow white miso

2 tablespoons tahini

1 tablespoon water

1–2 teaspoons agave syrup or other sweetener, optional

4 cups mixed greens

Combine the tamari, sesame oil and ginger in a medium bowl. Add the mushrooms and onions to the bowl and mix well to combine and coat the vegetables. Let sit for at least 15 minutes. Heat a grill pan or use the grill. Grill the mushrooms and onions until cooked through.

In a small bowl, combine the miso, tahini and water until smooth.

Put the washed greens in a bowl. Mix in the miso tahini dressing, and arrange on individual plates. Put the mushrooms and onions on top. Add freshly ground pepper, if desired.

Immune Broth

—JILL NUSSINOW—

I make a soup very similar to Tess Challis' "Immune Power Soup" called Immune Boosting Bowl. Rather than bore you with an almost identical soup, I'll share my recipe for the broth that I use for the soup. Two of the mushrooms that I use are not edible but add a lot to the broth. You will have to buy the dried mushrooms and astragalus at your local herb shop or online.

Makes 2 quarts

2–3 slices dried reishi mushroom

2–3 pieces dried turkey tail mushroom

1 large stick astragalus

3–4 dried shiitake mushrooms

2 cloves garlic, cut in half

1 1-inch piece ginger

1 small hot fresh or dried pepper, if desired

1 4-inch piece of kombu seaweed

8 cups water

Add the entire mixture to a soup pot and simmer for 30 minutes to 1 hour. Strain.

Or add to a pressure cooker and bring to high pressure over high heat. Reduce the heat to maintain high pressure for 5 minutes. Let the pressure come down naturally. Strain and use.

If you like, you can take out the rehydrated shiitake mushrooms and add them to your soup. Save the piece of kombu for your next batch of stock, or eat it. It helps soothe a sore throat.

Immune Power Soup

—TESS CHALLIS—

This soup is health in a bowl! It contains six medicinal superfoods that are sure to deliver. Shiitake mushrooms and kale are top notch foods for building strength and boosting the immune system. Miso is a powerful detoxifier and cleanser. Garlic is antibacterial and anticarcinogenic, and also helps to detoxify the body. Ginger treats colds and eases congestion. Dulse is strengthening and an excellent source of minerals. Knowing all of that, you can feel quite smug about eating this soup. Incidentally, I find that I can even get children to eat this by leaving (or picking!) out the shiitakes and scallions.

Serves 4

- 1 cup thinly sliced fresh or frozen shiitake mushroom caps
- 4 leaves of kale, de-stemmed and sliced into very thin ribbons
- 4 teaspoons each: toasted (dark) sesame oil and tamari, shoyu, or soy sauce
- ¼ cup dark (or red) miso
- 4 cups water, preferably filtered

- 4 medium to large cloves garlic, pressed or minced
- 4 teaspoons grated ginger (leave the peel on if organic), or more to taste
- 2 scallions (green onion), trimmed and minced
- 2 teaspoons dried dulse flakes (optional)

In a medium soup pot, sauté the shiitakes and kale in the oil and tamari for about 5 minutes over medium-low heat, stirring often. Remove from heat.

In a separate bowl, whisk a little of the water into the miso to create a smooth paste, being careful to stir out any lumps. A little at a time, whisk the remaining water into the miso, stirring well until very smooth.

Add the miso-water mixture to the soup pot and stir to combine. Add all of the remaining ingredients and stir well. Set to low heat and cook just until warmed through. Do not boil or overheat, as it can destroy many of the nutrients. Eat up and feel your batteries charge!

Mushroom Un–Meatballs

—JILL NUSSINOW—

This dish is quite simple to make. They look like meatballs but are full of mushroom flavor because they are almost all mushroom. The miso adds some salt and you can add freshly ground black pepper, too, if it suits you. I served them at a potluck and many of the vegetarians and vegans didn't eat them because they thought that they were made of meat.

Makes 24–36 depending upon the size

1 ounce mixed dried wild mushrooms, such as porcini or a mixed bag of them

5–6 dried shiitake mushrooms

1 tablespoon olive or other oil

½ medium onion, diced

5–6 ounces sliced crimini mushrooms

2 teaspoons tamari or soy sauce

3 tablespoons Italian parsley

2–3 cloves garlic

1 tablespoon mellow white miso

1 cup quick or baby rolled oats

1 tablespoon oil for sautéing un-meatballs

Soak dried mushrooms in hot water until they are pliable, 30 minutes to 1 hour. Drain the mushrooms,(saving the soaking water for a wonderful mushroom broth or soup) and roughly chop. Set mushrooms aside.

Heat the oil in a sauté pan over medium high heat. Add the onion and sauté for a minute or two. Add the sliced crimini mushrooms and sauté until they start browning and releasing some liquid, about 5–7 minutes. Add the rehydrated mushrooms and tamari. Sauté another few minutes until all the mushrooms seem cooked through and there is no liquid in the pan.

Pulse the cooked mushrooms in the food processor until they are finely chopped and put into a bowl.

In the same food processor, add the parsley and pulse until finely chopped. Add to the mushrooms. Pulse the garlic and then add the miso and pulse one more time. Add the miso and garlic to the mushrooms. Stir the oats into the mushrooms and mix well.

Let sit for a few minutes so that the oats can absorb some of the mushroom liquid. Form into balls about 1-inch in diameter. The mushroom mixture should be fairly dry and easy to work with. If you find that it's too sticky, you can add more oats.

Heat the remaining tablespoon oil over medium high heat. Add the un-meatballs in batches to the hot pan and brown on all sides. Serve warm.

Note: I made these in a nonstick pan and it worked really well. If I had more time, I might have made chutney to go with these meatballs or a sweet, sundried tomato "ketchup." You also can bake the "meatballs" on parchment in a 350°F oven for 15–20 minutes.

Simple Shiitake and Broccoli (Mock) Stir-Fry

—JILL NUSSINOW—

A traditional stir-fry uses a lot of oil. This one uses none. You want the mushrooms to be cooked through and for the broccoli to bright and crisp. The flavor of the mushrooms shines here.

Serves 4

8 ounces fresh shiitake mushrooms, sliced, stems removed and reserved for broth

4 cloves minced garlic

4 cups fresh broccoli florets

¼ cup or more vegetable broth

Freshly ground black pepper

½ teaspoon salt, optional

3 green onions, sliced on the diagonal

2 tablespoons sliced or slivered almonds, optional

Add the mushrooms and garlic over medium high heat in a large sauté pan. Dry sauté for 3–4 minutes, making sure that the garlic does not burn. Add the broccoli and the broth and cook for 2–3 more minutes until the broccoli is turning bright green. Cook until the mushrooms are done and the broccoli is cooked through. Add freshly ground black pepper, to taste and salt, if you desire. Put on a platter and sprinkle with the green onions and almonds.

Shiitake Mushroom Asparagus Spinach Soup

—KATJA HEINO—

Loaded with immune boosting shiitake mushrooms and vitamin and mineral rich spinach and asparagus, this delicious spring time soup makes for a nutrient-dense, satisfying meal the whole family will love. I use homemade nut milk to add a bit of creaminess to the soup, but feel free to use any dairy-free milk of your choice.

Serves 4–6

1 pound asparagus, ends trimmed off and cut into ½-inch pieces

2 cups shiitake mushrooms, fresh and chopped into thin slices

4 big handfuls of baby spinach, washed well and roughly chopped

1 small onion, finely chopped

4 cloves garlic, minced

4 cups homemade vegetable broth

½ teaspoon tarragon, dried

1 bay leaf

1 cup homemade nut milk of choice

¼ cup fresh parsley, finely chopped

juice of 1 lemon

salt and pepper, to taste

2 tablespoons coconut oil

Melt coconut oil in medium soup pot and sauté onion until translucent and beginning to brown. Add minced garlic and sauté for about a minute.

Add asparagus and shiitake mushrooms and sauté for 3–4 minutes until veggie start to sweat. Pour in 4 cups of broth and add bay leaf, tarragon, and spinach.

Simmer soup for about 30 minutes on low-medium heat until asparagus is nice and soft. Turn off heat, add nut milk, lemon juice and fresh parsley, cover and let sit on stove top for at least another 30 minutes (I usually let it sit for longer to let flavors meld)

Before serving, add salt and pepper to taste and reheat gently.

Tempeh and Wild Mushroom Stew

—JILL NUSSINOW—

Tempeh is a great way to get soy and is better for you than tofu as it's a whole food. Combined with mushrooms, it is a real winner. Steaming the tempeh opens it up to absorbing more flavor. You can also make it without the tempeh and if you love mushrooms, as I do, it is still delicious. Serve over your favorite whole grain.

Serves 4

- 1–2 ounces dried mushrooms such as porcini, morel or shiitake
- 1 cup water plus ½ cup water
- 8 ounces tempeh, cut into cubes
- 1 pound wild and regular mushrooms, any combination is fine
- 1 large red onion, chopped

- 2–3 teaspoons miso
- 1 tablespoon arrowroot
- 1 tablespoon fresh rosemary, chopped, or 1 teaspoon crumbled dried rosemary
- Freshly ground black pepper and salt, to taste

Boil the cup of water and soak the dried mushrooms, if they are morels or shiitake, for 30 minutes. Save the clean soaking water. If using porcini, add when recommended.

Steam the tempeh over boiling water for 15 minutes. Remove from heat and let cool.

Heat the sauté pan over medium heat. Add the onion and sauté for 3–5 minutes, until it starts to soften. Add the chopped wild mushrooms, the tempeh cubes and rosemary. Cook for about 7–8 minutes. Add the mushroom soaking water, drained of any debris or dirt, and the porcini, if using them. Add the miso and stir. Cook for another couple of minutes until the mushrooms are mostly cooked but do not boil so you keep the probiotic effect of the miso.

Combine the remaining ½ cup water with the arrowroot. Remove the pan from the heat, stir in the arrowroot mixture until well combined and then put back on the heat. If the mixture is too thick, add water 1 tablespoon at a time. If too thin, cook down or add 1 teaspoon arrowroot mixed with 1 tablespoon water until you achieve the desired consistency. Season with black pepper. Add salt to taste.

Wild Mushroom Ravioli

—JILL NUSSINOW—

These ravioli are simple to make with premade wonton or pot sticker wrappers. So far, I have not found a gluten-free version.

Serves 4-6 as an appetizer

1 tablespoon olive oil, optional

½ cup chopped shallots or onions

2 pounds assorted wild mushrooms such as shiitake, chanterelles, oyster or even some crimini (to cut the cost), finely chopped

1–2 teaspoons *Bragg Liquid Aminos* acids or tamari

½ (12.3-ounce) box *Mori-Nu* or 6 ounces other silken firm tofu

2 teaspoons mild miso

2 tablespoons chopped Italian parsley or cilantro

¼ teaspoon freshly ground pepper

1 package potsticker or wonton wrappers

Heat the oil in a sauté pan, if using, over medium heat. Add the shallots or onions and sauté for 3 minutes. Add the finely chopped mushrooms and sauté until the mushrooms start to release their juices. Continue to sauté until the mushrooms are fairly dry. Add the *Bragg Liquid Aminos* or tamari. Stir and remove from the heat.

Process the tofu in the food processor with the miso, parsley and pepper. Stir in the mushrooms.

Take 1 wrapper and place 2 tablespoons of filling on it. You can either fold over the wrapper and seal the edges with water, or if you want larger ravioli you can place another wrapper on top and seal the edges with water. Let sit only for a few minutes before putting into boiling water or they may get dried out. Cook the ravioli for 3–4 minutes, until the wrappers are cooked through.

Serve with a sauce, such as the "Rich Mushroom Gravy" page 126 on the side, or use a mushroom-based salad dressing or marinade.

Smoked Trumpet Mushroom Potato Soup

—JASON WYRICK—

I love mushrooms and I love working out on the grill. This recipe uses king trumpet (also called Trumpet Royale) mushrooms, which is a type of hearty and thick oyster mushroom. They stand up perfectly to the rigors of a rack and hot coals, and give the soup substance and crispy brown goodness. If you don't have a grill or it's the winter, you can roast these at 450°F in the oven until crispy.

Serves 2–3

- 4–5 Yukon gold or rose potatoes, chopped into large pieces
- 3 cups of veggie broth plus a bit more to replenish the broth as it cooks down
- 10 whole cloves of garlic
- ½ teaspoon salt
- 1 teaspoon smoked paprika
- ¾ teaspoon cracked black pepper
- 2 trumpet mushrooms (about 6 ounces), sliced into ¼-inch thick rounds
- ¼ teaspoon coarse sea salt (a large grain sel de gris works perfectly here)
- 1 tablespoon minced fresh flat leaf parsley

Chop the potatoes into large pieces (don't worry about getting this perfect since they are going to be puréed anyway; this just helps them cook faster). Simmer the potatoes and garlic in the veggie broth until the potatoes are soft (about 10 minutes). Replenish any evaporated veggie broth with more broth.

While the potatoes are simmering, get your grill lit. Spray a grill tray* with a few spritzes of oil. Slice the mushrooms and place them on a grill tray. Place the mushrooms directly over the hot part of the grill and stir them every minute or so until they are heavily browned on both sides. This can take from 8–12 minutes, depending on how hot your grill is and how close the rack is to the coals. Once they have developed dark brown areas along the ridges of the mushroom slices, remove them from the heat, toss them with the coarse sea salt, and set them to the side.

Purée the potatoes, garlic, salt, paprika, and pepper. Plate this in a shallow bowl and then add the grilled mushrooms. Top with fresh parsley.

---

*A grill tray has holes in the bottom. It is meant to sit on the rack in the grill. It allows you to hold quite a few smaller ingredients without them falling through the grill.

Trumpet Mushroom and Avocado Ceviche

—MIYOKO SCHINNER—

Very refreshing with a hint of the sea, it's perfect as a summer appetizer, or as an addition to tacos. While I recommend using trumpets as the primary mushroom for their meaty texture, you can use a variety of mushrooms to vary the texture and flavors.

Serves 6

12 ounces trumpet mushrooms, or combination of trumpet and other mushroom (such as shiitake, hedgehog, oyster)

½ red onion, sliced thinly, or 3–4 green onions, sliced

½ roasted red bell pepper, skinned, diced small

1 sheet nori, torn into little pieces

½ teaspoon cumin seeds

½ cup freshly squeezed lime juice

1 tablespoon sake

2 avocados, cubed

1 cup loosely packed cilantro

¼ cup loosely packed mint

Salt and pepper to taste

Clean the mushrooms by wiping with a damp cloth. Cut them into bite-sized pieces, or slice into ¼-inch slices. Don't make them too small, because they will shrink, and you want meaty pieces to chew on.

Put them into a medium bowl, and combine with the nori, roasted red bell pepper, cumin seeds, lime juice, and sake. Cover, and refrigerate for 2–3 hours to marinate. Gently toss with the avocado, cilantro, and mint, and season with salt and pepper to taste. Serve chilled.

Mushroom Oat Burgers

—JILL NUSSINOW—

Vegetables form the basis of this burger. The oats give them a nice crunch. They are similar to a popular commercially prepared veggie burger but, of course, these are all plant-based.

Serves 4

Vegetable cooking spray or spray oil, optional

1 cup chopped onion

⅓ pound white, crimini or shiitake mushrooms, sliced to equal about 1½ cups

½ cup chopped broccoli

1 medium carrot, grated to equal ½ cup

3 cloves garlic, minced

¼ cup chopped roasted red pepper

¾ cup cooked brown rice

1 tablespoon egg replacer mixed with ¼ cup water or 2 tablespoons flaxseeds, ground and mixed with ¼ cup water

½ cup grated non-dairy mozzarella cheese

1¾ cups rolled oats, divided

½ teaspoon pepper

Salt to taste

Spray a nonstick sauté pan with cooking spray, if using. Add onion and cook over medium heat for 3 minutes. Add the mushrooms, broccoli, carrot and garlic and sauté for another 2 minutes. Cover pan and cook for another 5 minutes. Remove from heat and put vegetable mixture in a medium bowl. Rinse pan for later use.

Let vegetables cool slightly, and put in a food processor with roasted red pepper, brown rice and egg replacer mixture or flax and water. Process for 15–30 seconds until the mixture still has some texture but no large chunks. Add the cheese and 1 cup of the oats and process for another 10 seconds, pulsing on and off. Empty processor contents into a large bowl and combine with the remaining oats, salt and pepper, stirring thoroughly. The burger mixture will be a bit wet, but will firm up considerably with cooking. Form into 8 patties 3-inches in diameter and ¾-inch thick.

Spray the pan with cooking spray. Add the patties to the pan and cook over medium heat for 5 minutes. Flip burgers and cook 5 more minutes.

If you prefer, you can bake the burgers at 350°F. on a parchment lined baking sheet for 10 minutes. Turn and bake the other side until crisp. Serve on buns with traditional toppings.

Note: After cooking, these burgers may be refrigerated or frozen and thawed. They can then be warmed through in a toaster oven or on the grill.

C H A M P S

Pulses Included

Adzuki Beans

Black Beans

Black-Eyed Peas

Chickpeas or Garbanzo Beans

Kidney Beans

Lentils

Mung Beans

Peas

Pinto Beans

Soybeans

Split Peas

White Beans

Yellow Eyed Beans

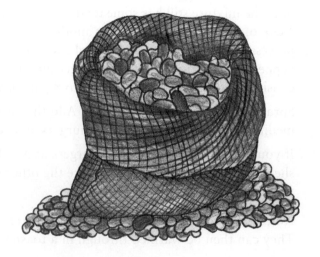

CHAPTER 5

Pulses:
Beans, Lentils and Peas

WHETHER YOU CALL THEM pulses, legumes or beans, peas and lentils, this category of food is undeniably the foundation for plant-based eating, providing amazing nutrition, answering that all-too-often-asked question, "Where do you get your protein?"

Legumes are nature's answer to providing variety, taste, texture, shape and color on your plate. There are hundreds, if not thousands, of varieties of heirloom beans. Here we have stuck mostly to the standard varieties but I would be remiss if I didn't tell you that you can expand your horizon beyond those in these recipes. (Read "Lovely Legumes: Full of Beans" on page 148 and the "Ingredient Sources" section on pages 244-245.)

You might be thinking, "I can't afford to buy those pricey legumes..." I want you to know that even at five to seven dollars a pound, you are getting maximum nutrition for your dollars spent. One pound of beans usually yields 6–7 servings. No other protein food can compare to this.

In addition to protein, beans contain complex carbohydrates, soluble fiber, which keeps their glycemic index low, magnesium, copper and iron, among other minerals. They also contain B vitamins. These nutrients have been shown to improve lipid profiles, helping to lower your cholesterol, and to improve insulin sensitivity which helps regulate blood sugar.

Studies have shown that including 1 cup of beans per day for Type 2 Diabetics can improve hemoglobin A1c values as well as decreasing the calculated risk for coronary heart disease and reducing systolic blood pressure.[1]

A recent study found that the consumption of beans was the most valuable predictor of survival in various ethnicities in people older than seventy.[2] No other food group had this effect. I can't think of a better reason to eat beans except that I enjoy eating them so much.

---

[1] Arch Intern Med. 2012;172(21):1653-1660
[2] Asia Pac J Clin Nutr. 2004;13(2):217-20

Lovely Legumes: Full of Beans

Beans, peas and lentils have gone from peasant fare to upscale, found at expensive restaurants and gourmet stores. The range of available pulses or legumes, which is what they are called, is amazing. You'll find tiny black Beluga lentils, just a fraction of an inch round, to Christmas lima or scarlet runner beans, at a full inch or two long. Each legume looks different and can be used in a myriad of recipes from appetizers through dessert.

I praise beans for their versatility and variety, however their taste holds the allure. If you've tried limas and didn't like them (most people say they don't until they taste them), then try garbanzo, also known as chickpea, or kidney beans, or green (edamame), yellow or black soybeans. The range of colors seen in beans is astounding.

Beans that have been in existence for a long time are called "heirloom" beans. While grown from "old" stock, they are usually more recently harvested. Old beans will not completely cook through and are often tough. Buying beans at a natural food store rather than in a bag at the supermarket will often yield a newer crop of beans. And a specialty bean purveyor will have the freshest (see the "Ingredient Sources" section on pages 244-245).

Tierra Vegetables' farm stand in Santa Rosa, California sells a bean called Marrow Fat. It's so creamy and delicious that it has been added to the Slow Foods Ark of Taste, to be preserved for future generations.

Just a sampling of other terrific tasting heirlooms includes Anasazi, borlotti, flageolet, Jacob's cattle, and yellow eye Stueben. There are so many legume varieties to explore that you could try one a week for a year or more.

Eating beans often seems to help your body adjust to beans and decreases gas. If that doesn't work, you try adding kombu seaweed when cooking beans. Or you can sprout your beans for two to three days, rinsing two to three times a day and storing in the dark, before you drain and cook them. They generally will then only need half the cooking time. Do not add salt or other acidic foods such as tomatoes or molasses during cooking or else your beans may be tough. To boost flavor, add herbs, spices or garlic to your bean pot or pressure cooker. (See the article "The Pressure Cooker and Pulses Can Save Your Life or at Least Your Time" on page 188 for more information about pressure cookers).

There's an old saying, "Beans, beans, good for your heart..." Protect your heart today in a tasty way.

—Jill Nussinow

Asian-Adzuki Bean Crockpot Chili

—JL FIELDS—

This simple to put together dish pairs two of my favorite foods: adzuki beans and winter squash which mingle to form a wonderfully easy one-pot dish.

Serves 4–6

2 tablespoons olive oil

1 packet concentrated low-sodium vegetable broth (I used *Trader Joe's Savory Broth Liquid Concentrate*)

1 (15-ounce) can fire roasted diced tomatoes

2½ (15-ounce) cans of water

1 tablespoon double-concentrate tomato paste

2 large cloves of garlic

2 carrots, diced

1 small onion

1½ cups adzuki beans (dry, and no, I did not soak them)

½ teaspoon *Herbamare* (or sea salt)

2 teaspoon Sriracha

1 tablespoon *Bragg Liquid Aminos* or low-sodium soy sauce

½ teaspoon dulse flakes (optional)

2 cups cabbage, diced

Add all ingredients to the crockpot and cook on high for 5 hours. Add cabbage 3 hours into cooking. Serve hot.

Protein Powerhouse Trifecta

—ELLEN JONES—

Vegan athletes cringe when they hear the too frequently-asked question, "Where do you get your protein?" But probably a day doesn't go by when we do. It is always an opportunity to educate, no matter how tired we may be of answering it. Eating plant-based proteins have served many athletes well in all kinds of sports. But even if you're not training for a marathon, a serving of this protein-rich bean and nut entrée will keep your muscles in tip-top shape for whatever events you have planned. Quinoa has more protein than any other whole grain.

Serves 6–8

¼ cup vegetable broth

4 cloves garlic, minced

1 medium yellow onion, chopped

2 tablespoons low-salt soy sauce or tamari

1 tablespoon balsamic vinegar

1 bunch kale, stems removed, rolled and cut in thin strips

1 cup cooked adzuki beans

1 tablespoon miso, dissolved in 2 tablespoons warm but not boiling hot water

3 cups cooked quinoa

4 tablespoons raw sunflower seeds

In a large pot or wok, add the garlic and onion to the vegetable broth and cook over medium heat until both are translucent. Add the soy sauce, vinegar and kale. Cook the kale until it is just soft.

Add the adzuki beans and warm thoroughly. Turn off the heat, and then add the miso. Use a spoon or spatula to turn the kale leaves over, blending well the miso and other ingredients.

Spoon servings over the quinoa. Sprinkle with the sunflower seeds.

Black Bean and Greens Quesadillas
with Smoky Chipotle Cream

—JENN LYNSKEY—

This dish is adapted from the Mayan Quesadilla that I ordered religiously at Tijuana Taxi in Rehoboth Beach, Delaware. The original featured spinach and a thick rich chipotle mayo and was my first taste of the smoky spicy concoction. The restaurant is no longer in business, but my love of chipotles has certainly lived on! Chipotles are widely available in most grocery stores, but the chipotle sauce is flexible and you can use a canned chipotle pepper, a dried whole chipotle that has been rehydrated in hot water, or dried chipotle powder depending on what you can easily find.

Serves 4

FILLING

¼ cup water

1 small sweet onion cut in half and sliced thinly

½ teaspoon oregano

Pinch salt

1 cup cooked black beans

2 cups packed chopped greens of your choice

SPICY CHIPOTLE SAUCE

1 cup soft silken tofu

1 chipotle pepper in adobe or rehydrated or 1 teaspoon dried chipotle powder

Juice of 1 lime

¼ cup packed fresh cilantro

Pinch salt to taste

8 corn or small whole wheat tortillas

In a small food processor or blender, add tofu, chipotle, lime juice, cilantro, and salt. Blend until smooth.

In a sauté pan add water, onions, oregano, and salt and cook until onion is translucent. Add beans and greens then cover and cook until beans are heated and greens are wilted.

Heat a cast iron skillet over medium heat. Place one tortilla on the dry skillet and add ¼ of filling evenly over tortilla leaving space at the edges (looks like a pizza with crust around the edge.) Then add another tortilla to top. Cook 1 minute, then flip and cook 1 minute more. Repeat with remaining tortillas and filling. Cut into 8 pieces (again similar to a pizza) and serve topped with chipotle sauce with additional cilantro to garnish.

Black Bean and Sweet Potato Hash

—JILL NUSSINOW—

This is an ideal breakfast food for me but others will probably like it for lunch or a light dinner. It can be served over brown rice or quinoa, wrapped in a whole wheat tortilla or made into a soft taco, or as a side dish.

Serves 4

1 tablespoon oil, optional

1 cup chopped onion

1–2 cloves garlic, minced

2 cups chopped sweet potatoes, about 2 small to medium, peeled

2 teaspoons chili powder (not spice)

½ cup vegetable broth

¼ teaspoon salt

1 cup cooked black beans

¼ cup green onion, chopped

Splash of hot sauce, to taste

Salt to taste

Cilantro, chopped for garnish

Heat the oil in a sauté pan over medium high heat. Add the onion and sauté for 2–3 minutes. Add the garlic for another minute. Then add the sweet potatoes and chili powder. Stir to coat the sweet potatoes with chili. Add the vegetable broth and stir. Cover the pan, lower the heat to medium and cook for 8 minutes, stirring occasionally.

Remove the lid and add the salt, black beans and green onion. Cook another minute or two, until the beans are heated through. Add hot sauce, if desired. Taste and add more salt, if you like. Top with chopped cilantro.

Black Bean Collard Wraps

—MORGAN ECCLESTON—

Collard greens make a wonderful alternative to tortillas for wraps. I like to use the biggest fresh collards that I can find for these. For a spicy smoky kick you can add 1–2 minced chipotle peppers to the filling.

Serves 4 (2 rolls per serving)

- 2 (15-ounce) cans black beans drained (about 3 cups)
- 1 cup cooked brown rice
- ½ red pepper, chopped
- 2 green onions, chopped
- 1 jalapeno, minced
- 3 cloves garlic, minced
- ¼ teaspoon kosher salt
- 1 teaspoon hot sauce
- 8 large fresh collard greens, washed and stems removed (keep the top of the leaf intact)

Prepare a steamer for the collard greens. Steam them for 2–3 minutes or until pliable. Set aside.

Mash the black beans and cooked rice together in a large bowl. Add in remaining ingredients and mix thoroughly. Warm in a large pan over medium high heat until warmed through.

Overlap the edges of the greens and put about ½ cup of the filling in the middle. Fold in the edges of the collard and roll up the filling like a burrito. Continue with the rest of the greens and filling.

Black Bean Peanut Butter Brownies

—HEATHER NICHOLDS—

These brownies are sweetened with banana and fresh dates, although I do have an option to make them with unrefined sugar if you prefer. The rich, fudgy base comes from a combo of kidney beans, peanut butter and cocoa powder, so you don't need any oil to make these. I've fallen in love with sorghum flour, thanks to Allyson Kramer of ManifestVegan.com, and it works perfectly in these brownies to leave them gluten-free. If you can't find sorghum, you can use buckwheat, brown rice, spelt or even whole wheat flour. The downside of whole wheat is that it tastes a bit heavy, and makes the batter really sticky. However you make them, though, they're moist and chocolatey and so delicious no one will ever guess that they're also super healthy.

Makes 16 brownies

1 (15-ounce) can black or kidney beans

1 banana

½ cup fresh medjool dates, pitted*

½ cup non-dairy milk

½ cup natural peanut butter (or any other nut/seed butter)

1 teaspoon vanilla extract

1 teaspoon apple cider vinegar

1 teaspoon baking powder

½ teaspoon baking soda

¾ cup cocoa and/or carob powder

½ cup raisins, dried cranberries or chocolate chips (or a mix of any or all)

1 cup sorghum flour (or any whole grain flour)

Preheat the oven to 400°F (or your BBQ on low, about 450°F).

Put the beans, banana, dates, milk, nut/seed butter, vanilla and apple cider vinegar in a food processor and purée until smooth. If you don't have a food processor, you can mash the beans and banana, and chop the dates up as finely as you can. The sweetness won't be as even as if you purée, so you may want to add some unrefined sugar.

Add the baking powder, soda, cocoa/carob powder and flour and pulse until they're incorporated. Don't overmix here. Sprinkle the raisins, cranberries or chocolate chips into the mix and push them into the batter (don't purée them).

Pour the batter into a greased or lined 8-inch brownie dish and put in the oven for 30–40 minutes. Once the brownies are cooked, pull them from the oven, let them cool completely and then cut into squares and serve. If you want to keep your brownies longer, they freeze very well.

---

* If you prefer, or if you're not using a food processor, you can replace the dates with ½ cup unrefined sugar.

Brazilian Black Bean Stew *(Feijoada)*

—LYDIA GROSSOV—

Feijoada is a traditional dish Brazilians love eating for lunch on a Friday. This plant-based version is packed with protein, iron, fiber, tons of flavor and no cholesterol. Serve it with a side of brown rice, collard greens sautéed with garlic and some orange wedges.

Serves 4–6

1 teaspoon extra virgin olive oil or 1 tablespoon of water

1 yellow onion

6 garlic cloves, thinly sliced

1 medium-sized eggplant, cubed

2 tablespoons water

1 pound sliced assorted mushrooms: crimini, stemmed shiitake and maitake (hen of the woods)

1 tablespoon of low-sodium gluten-free tamari

2 (29-ounce) cans low sodium, organic black beans or fresh cooked, undrained beans to equal about 6 cups

1½ cups of water

1 teaspoon salt or to taste

1 teaspoon fresh ground pepper

4 bay leaves

Place the olive oil, onion and garlic in a stock pot and sauté for 2–3 minutes. For oil-free, sauté them with water or dry sauté and add water, as needed.

Add the cubed eggplant and 2 tablespoons of water. Cook for 5 minutes over medium heat with the lid on.

Add the mushroom medley and tamari. Cook for an additional 5–8 minutes, until most of the liquid from the mushrooms have cooked down and the eggplant is tender.

Add the black beans, remaining water, salt, pepper and bay leaves and simmer for 10 minutes to heat through and incorporate all of the flavors. Adjust salt and pepper to taste if necessary.

Spicy Black Bean Dip

—JILL NUSSINOW—

You can use this dip to make veggies more interesting or you can use as a spread for wraps. I have even taken the dip and mixed it with cooked grains to make quick and tasty burgers.

Makes about 2 cups

1 can black beans, drained or
  2 cups cooked

2–3 cloves garlic, pressed

1 teaspoon cumin powder

2 teaspoons chili powder

1 dash of cayenne pepper

2 teaspoons chopped onion

1 tablespoon lime juice

1 tablespoon *Bragg Liquid Aminos*
  or tamari

4 tablespoons minced cilantro, save
  1 for garnish

Combine all ingredients except 1 tablespoon cilantro into the food processor. If the mixture seems too thick, add water 1 tablespoon at a time until it is the desired consistency.

Easy Salsa Supper

—ELISA RODRIGUEZ—

This dish is easy to prepare, quick to assemble, and it allows you to personalize the ingredients based on your preference. It's delicious, satisfying, and full of nutrients. Use whole grains such as teff, millet, brown rice, quinoa, or barley. Try a new leafy green such as mustard or turnip greens, kale, collards, Swiss chard, or bok choy. Vary your bean selection with black beans, white canellini beans, chick peas, black-eyed peas, chili beans, butter beans, or a mix. Choose your favorite salsa to top it off!

Serves 2–4

1 onion, chopped

1–2 cups mango salsa (or any salsa of your choice)

2 cups quinoa (or any whole grain)

1–2 cups black-eyed peas (or any bean variety, or cubed tofu)

1 bunch of kale (or any leafy green)

2 tablespoons sherry (optional)

1–2 avocados (½ per person)

Fresh cilantro to garnish

Cook your whole grain of choice on the stove top. Meanwhile cut your onion and prepare your greens.

Sauté the onion and salsa in a large skillet over medium heat. Add the beans or well-drained tofu to the skillet. Add the greens and allow them to soften. Add the cooked whole grain of choice. Add the sherry if the salsa dries up and begins to stick at any time, or add it in with the grains for additional flavor as desired. Stir the ingredients together well. Turn off the heat and allow the flavors to set in for a couple minutes.

Serve with cubed avocado on top, about ½ avocado per person. Garnish with fresh cilantro.

Fresh Shelling Beans and Summer Vegetables

—JILL NUSSINOW—

You can use any fresh bean that you can buy. Locally we can get black-eyed peas, marrow fat, cranberry, scarlett runner and others. The season is short. They cook quickly and go well with any other summer vegetables. I like to add toasted cumin for the best flavor.

Serves 4

½ cup diced onion

2–3 cloves garlic

½ cup diced colored pepper

2–3 teaspoons hot pepper, if desired

2–3 teaspoons toasted cumin

1½ to 2 cups shelled beans

¼ cup vegetable stock

¼ cup diced tomatillo

½ cup diced tomato

½ cup fresh corn, if desired

Dry sauté the onion for 2 minutes. Add the garlic and pepper. Sauté another minute. Add the cumin, beans and stock. Lock the lid on the pressure cooker and cook for 2 minutes. Quick release the pressure. Add the tomatillo, tomato and corn, if you are using it. Sauté for a few minutes until the tomato starts to break down. Serve hot.

You can easily do this on the stove top but will likely need more liquid. Make sure that the beans are cooked through before adding the tomatillo, tomato and corn. It will take about 10 minutes total, although each batch of beans is different.

Smoky Sweet Black-Eyed Peas

—JILL NUSSINOW—

I love black-eyed peas and I don't just reserve them for New Year's luck. Any day that I can eat them is a lucky day.

Serves 4–6

1 teaspoon oil, optional

1 medium to large onion, thinly sliced

2–3 cloves garlic, minced

1 cup diced red pepper

1 small jalapeno or other hot chile, minced

1–2 teaspoons smoked paprika

1–2 teaspoons chili powder

1½ cups dried black-eyed peas, soaked overnight and drained

4 dates, chopped fine

3 cups water plus more as needed

1 (15-ounce) can Fire Roasted tomatoes with green chilies

2 cups chopped greens such as kale, collards or Swiss chard

Salt to taste

Heat a large saucepan over medium heat. Dry sauté the onion for a few minutes, adding some of the water if the onion starts to stick. Add the garlic and peppers and sauté for another minute. Add the smoked paprika and chili powder along with the peas and dates. Stir to coat them and then add the water to cover them. Bring to a boil and reduce the heat to a simmer. Put a lid on, keeping it slightly ajar. Cook by simmering, keeping the peas covered with water, for 35–45 minutes until they are cooked through and almost all of the water has been absorbed. Drain any excess water.

Add the tomatoes and greens and cook for another 5 minutes or more until the greens are wilted. Add salt to taste.

Note: The pea mixture can be pressure cooked up until the point where you add the tomatoes. It will require 1½ cups water, under pressure for just 3 minutes with a natural pressure release. You can add the tomatoes and greens and pressure cook for 1 more minute, or simmer on the stove top for a few minutes.

Chickpea Curry

—VICTORIA MORAN—

I've been lucky enough to visit India on two occasions. Every time I make a curry, it takes me back.

Serves 4–6

2 tablespoons olive oil, coconut oil, vegetable broth or cooking wine

1 teaspoon coriander

1 teaspoon cumin

1 ¼ teaspoon turmeric

¼ teaspoon ground cloves

¼ teaspoon cinnamon

2 large cloves garlic, minced

⅛ teaspoon cayenne

1 pound green beans cut into 1-inch pieces

1 pound potatoes (Yellow Finn are lovely), peeled and cubed

2 medium carrots, thinly sliced

2 cups water

1 teaspoon salt

1 (20-ounce) can chickpeas (garbanzos), drained or 2 cups cooked

Heat oil on medium flame until hot (but not smoking). Add all seasonings except salt and cook for 2 minutes. Add the beans, potatoes, and carrots, and mix well. Add water and salt and heat to the boiling point. Reduce to low, and cook, covered, for 15 minutes. Add chickpeas and simmer until the liquid reduces by half. Serve over rice and accompany with a lovely chutney, in the Indian section of your supermarket.

Basmati is fragrant, long-grained rice that's perfect with Indian cuisine; you can purchase either.

Chickpea and Strawberry Summer Salad

—JAIME KARPOVICH—

When strawberries are in season in the summer, this makes an unusual but very tasty salad.

Serves 4–6

1 cup sliced strawberries

3 cups cooked chickpeas

Juice of 2 medium lemons

About ⅓ cup chopped flat leaf parsley

1 bunch scallions/green onions, chopped

¼ cup red onion, diced small

1–2 tablespoons dried mint

Sea salt and fresh cracked pepper to taste

Slice strawberries into thin rounds and add to a large mixing bowl with chickpeas. Pour lemon juice into the bowl and mix to coat. Add remaining ingredients and mix together.

I love to make this quick tomato soup for dinner when I need to get something on the table in a hurry. You can substitute ¼ cup of minced fresh basil for the mint, if you desire.

Chickpea Tomato Soup

—MORGAN ECCLESTON—

This semi-chunky soup comes together in a flash. You'll likely make this over and over again. You can also cook your own beans if you prefer.

Serves 6

½ large onion, chopped

1 carrot, chopped

1 stalk celery, chopped

¼ teaspoon kosher salt

1 clove garlic, minced

3 (14-ounce) cans diced tomatoes

2 cans chickpeas (garbanzo beans), drained (about 3 cups)

2 cups low sodium vegetable stock

1 tablespoon fresh rosemary, minced fine

2 tablespoons balsamic vinegar

Freshly ground black pepper to taste

Sauté the onion, carrot and celery with 2 tablespoons of water in a large pot over high heat until the onions are translucent. Add the salt and minced garlic. Stir and cook one minute longer.

Add in the tomatoes, 1 can (1½ cups) of chickpeas, vegetable stock and rosemary. Bring to a boil and then turn down to low heat and cover. Let simmer for 15 minutes.

Purée the soup with an immersion blender until very smooth (or in a regular blender in batches.) Add in the remaining can of chickpeas and heat until warmed through. Stir in the balsamic vinegar and add black pepper to taste.

Falafel Patties

—LESLIE CERIER—

Here's a delicious, easy to make, vegetarian and gluten-free recipe of this traditional Middle Eastern dish. Serve on a bed a salad or stuffed into pita pockets with a tahini dressing for a great lunch or dinner. Makes a great appetizer, too. Enjoy!

Serves 4 (1 dozen patties)

2 cups garbanzo bean flour

1 cup coarsely chopped cilantro

½ cup onions, coarsely chopped

½ cup water

3 cloves garlic, coarsely chopped or minced

2 tablespoons lemon juice

1 teaspoon cumin seeds

1 teaspoon *Celtic Sea Salt®*

3 tablespoons ghee or extra virgin coconut oil

Place all the ingredients, except the ghee or oil in a mixing bowl, and mix well. Shape the batter into walnut sized balls. Heat a 9-inch skillet. Add ghee or oil. Add falafel balls when oil is hot and flatten with a spatula. Fry on both sizes until golden brown. Serve on top of salad or stuffed into pita.

Variation: Swap 1 teaspoon ground coriander for cilantro.

Greek Garbanzo Bean Salad

—JILL NUSSINOW—

I like chickpeas or garbanzo beans in every form. This one combines some of my favorite flavors and is very easy to make.

Serves 6

3 cups garbanzo beans, cooked or canned

6 sundried tomatoes, rehydrated and chopped

2 tablespoons kalamata olives, chopped

1 cup cooked orzo pasta or cooked quinoa

¼ cup thinly sliced red onions

3 tablespoons lemon juice

2 tablespoons extra virgin olive oil, optional

1 teaspoon dried or 1 tablespoon fresh oregano

2 tablespoons chopped fresh Italian parsley

Salt and freshly ground black pepper to taste

Combine all the ingredients in a large bowl. Chill for at least 15 minutes. Taste and adjust the seasoning, add more lemon juice, salt or pepper, to taste.

Hummus

—JILL NUSSINOW—

No vegetarian book would be complete without a recipe for hummus. It's easily adaptable (add spinach, roasted red pepper, olives or whatever you like) and easy to make. Using canned beans makes it as quick as a trip to the store. Why buy it at the store when you can flavor anyway that you like at home? It's a great dip or sandwich spread and can be made into salad dressing. At least that's what one of my students told me. This is good served with warmed pita bread triangles or raw vegetables. Sometimes I put it in pita bread with salad and eat it for a sandwich.

Serves 6 as an appetizer

2 cloves garlic

1½ to 2 cups cooked garbanzo
  beans, you may use canned

2 tablespoons sesame tahini

2 tablespoons fresh lemon juice

½ teaspoon ground cumin

1 dash of cayenne pepper

1 tablespoon reduced sodium tamari
  or *Bragg Liquid Aminos*

2–4 tablespoons water

Put garlic in food processor to be sure that it gets well chopped. Whir for about 15 seconds. Add the remaining ingredients, blending until it's the desired consistency. If it seems too thick, add more water or bean cooking liquid or lemon juice.

Kidney Bean Salad
with Chili-Lime Dressing

—JOANNE WILLIAMS—

With hearty kidney beans, creamy avocados, crunchy fresh corn and a tasty chili-lime dressing, no one will suspect that this delicious salad is also rich in protein, high in fiber and perfect for those who avoid meat, dairy and gluten. And it couldn't be any easier to prepare!

Serves 4

DRESSING

2 tablespoons freshly squeezed lime juice

1 tablespoon cold-pressed hemp oil

¼ teaspoon ground cumin

¼ teaspoon ground chili powder

¼ teaspoon salt, or to taste

Freshly ground black pepper to taste

SALAD

2 cans kidney beans, drained and rinsed

Kernels from 2 large ears corn

1 red bell pepper, diced (about 1 cup)

1 avocado, diced

½ cup diced red onion

Place dressing ingredients in a large bowl and whisk until well combined. Add all salad ingredients and gently toss until evenly coated with dressing.

Refrigerate until ready to serve.

Vegan Red Beans and Rice

—ELLEN KANNER—

Red beans and rice is a New Orleans tradition, where they call it RBR. They serve it up every Monday, alas often with meat. This plant-based version gets its rich smoky flavor from smoked paprika and slow cooking. The beans need to be soaked overnight beforehand. Plan ahead. Ladle over rice — white rice is traditional in New Orleans, brown is healthier. Keep the hot sauce handy.

Serves 6 generously *(the way red beans and rice is supposed to be served)*

1 pound dried red beans (aka kidney beans), picked over, rinsed and soaked overnight

6 cups water

8 garlic cloves, 2 whole, 6 chopped

3 bay leaves

3 tablespoons olive oil

2 large onions, chopped

5 stalks celery, chopped

2 red or green peppers, chopped

2 teaspoons fresh thyme leaves from a few sprigs of thyme or 1 teaspoon dried thyme

2 teaspoons of your favorite hot sauce (more if you like it hot)

1 teaspoon allspice

2 teaspoons smoked paprika

1 dried pepper, crumbled or pinch red pepper flakes (optional)

Generous amount of sea salt and fresh ground pepper to taste

Rinse and drain soaked beans.

Bring 6 cups of water to boil in a large soup pot. Throw in two whole garlic cloves, 1 bay leaf and the optional dried pepper. Add the beans. Cover and reduce heat to medium. Leave the beans to themselves for 2 hours, or until tender but shapely.

In a separate large pot, heat the oil over medium-high heat. Add the 6 cloves chopped garlic, the chopped onions, celery and peppers. Cook, stirring, until vegetables soften and glisten with the oil, about 10 minutes. Add the thyme, hot sauce, allspice and smoked paprika and optional and dried pepper. Carefully tip the beans into the pot of vegetables. Stir to combine.

Bring to a boil, then reduce heat to medium or medium-low, until you reach a very low simmer. Continue cooking, uncovered for 2–3 hours. The longer it cooks, the happier the beans and you will be. You need only give it an occasional stir.

When you have a pot of creamy red and you can't tell where the beans start and the vegetables end, you have achieved RBR.

Remove bay and whole garlic cloves. Season with sea salt and pepper.

Lemony Lentil and Potato Chowder

—JILL NUSSINOW—

I love lentils and the red ones break down so nicely but unfortunately turn yellow when cooked. This is comfort food at its best. The lemon and mint also makes it incredibly refreshing and fresh tasting, something not always easy to do mid-winter.

Serves 6–8

1 tablespoon olive oil, optional

1 medium onion, sliced

1 tablespoon minced garlic

¼ teaspoon cayenne pepper

2 cups red lentils

6 cups vegetable broth

3 cups unpeeled diced potatoes (red look nice but any will work)

1 cup chopped greens like kale, mustard, chard, collards or sorrel

1 teaspoon lemon zest

4 tablespoons lemon juice

¼ cup chopped mint

Salt and freshly ground black pepper, to taste

Heat the oil, if using, over medium heat in a large stockpot. Add onion and sauté for 3–4 minutes until it begins to soften. Stir in the garlic and cayenne and cook for 1 minute more. Add the lentils, broth and potatoes. Bring the mixture to a boil, then reduce to a simmer.

Simmer, covered, for about 25 minutes or until the lentils and potatoes are tender. Purée the mixture with a hand blender. Add the greens and cook 5 more minutes until they are wilted.

Stir in the lemon zest and juice and the mint. Add salt and pepper, to taste.

Curried Lentils and Spinach

—JILL NUSSINOW—

Lentils like many other legumes are chameleons. They are traditionally used in Indian cooking. Serve this on top of brown rice or another favorite grain.

Serves 4

2 teaspoons canola or other neutral oil, optional

1 medium onion, diced

2 cloves garlic, minced

1 teaspoon grated ginger root or ½ teaspoon powdered ginger

1½ teaspoons curry powder

½ teaspoon cumin seeds

Pinch of cayenne pepper, if desired

1¼ cups brown or green lentils

2 cups vegetable broth

1 (10-ounce) package frozen spinach, thawed and drained

1 tablespoon lemon juice

Salt and pepper, to taste

Cilantro or mint, for garnish

Heat the oil in a medium (1½ to 2 quart) saucepan over medium heat. Add the onion and sauté for 2–3 minutes. Add the garlic and sauté for 30 seconds, then add the ginger, curry powder, cumin seeds and cayenne, if using. Sauté another 30 seconds and then add the lentils and stock.

Bring to a boil, then reduce to a simmer. Simmer for 30 minutes and test to see if lentils are cooked through. When the lentils are close to being thoroughly cooked, add the spinach and cook until hot.

Remove from the heat, add the lemon juice. Taste and add salt and pepper. Top with chopped cilantro or mint.

Lentil Coconut Spinach Soup

—JUDITH KINGSBURY—

Thick, rich warming curried lentil soup recipe, adapted from a recipe on Traveler's Lunchbox. Many thanks!! Green lentils were specified in the Traveler's Lunchbox version, but I've used both brown and French lentils with good effect, and I think they have better flavor. This can also be made on the stove top (with no pressure cooker) but it will take much longer, about 30 minutes.

Serves 6

1 cup brown or French lentils

2¼ cups water or unsalted vegetable stock

1 small kohlrabi, peeled and chopped in ½-inch dice (approximately 1 cup)

1 medium carrot, halved lengthwise and sliced thin

1 stalk celery, sliced thin

1-inch strip dried kombu seaweed, optional

1 bay leaf

½ teaspoon dried thyme leaf

1 teaspoon olive oil

1 cup minced onion, and 1–2 cloves minced garlic, optional

½ teaspoon smoked paprika

1 teaspoon curry powder, mild or hot, to your taste

4 cups coarsely chopped spinach leaves, or 6 cups baby spinach

½ can light coconut milk

2 tablespoons fresh lime juice

¼ teaspoon salt or to taste

Fresh ground pepper to taste

Wash lentils and soak 4 hours or more in cold lightly salted water.

Drain and cook lentils with 2¼ cups water, seaweed and bay leaf for 5 minutes at high pressure, natural pressure release. When the pressure indicator goes down, remove kombu strip and bay leaf from the lentils.

Chop vegetables as specified in ingredient list. Heat oil on medium in a sauté pan or large fry pan.

Sauté minced onion and garlic for 2 minutes, if using, until transparent.

Add chopped kohlrabi, carrot and celery. Sauté 2 minutes. Add curry powder, paprika and thyme. Stir for another minute. Add 2 tablespoons water and stir to release all the good bits from the bottom of the pan.

Then stir vegetable spice mixture into the lentils in the pressure cooker, lock the lid and bring to high pressure. Lower heat and cook for 3 minutes, with quick pressure release.

Stir in 1 cup light coconut milk and lime juice Add spinach to the soup. Stir on medium heat until spinach is wilted Add salt and pepper, adjust seasonings to taste

Cooking Tips:

I always cook double the amount of lentils, and freeze half so I can make lentil soup some other day. Or you could double the whole recipe and freeze half for take along meals.

If you can't find kohlrabi or don't enjoy it, fennel or cauliflower are both very good in this soup.

Make this soup almost fat free by combining the veggies and spices with the lentils, without sautéing in oil first, or use a water sauté method.

If you need to use salted soup stock, eliminate the added salt and kombu, so your soup won't be overly salty.

This is a thick main dish soup, almost a stew. You can expand it by adding more water or stock or coconut milk to make a thinner soup, and adjust seasonings to taste.

Lentil-Leek Soup

—JOANNE WILLIAMS—

Vegetarians are often asked, "Where do you get your protein?" A good answer would be, "Lentils!" Besides being rich in protein they are also a good source of dietary fiber, folate (important during pregnancy), iron, and other critical nutrients. This soup provides an impressive 15 grams of protein and 19 grams of dietary fiber.

Serves 4

2 teaspoons extra-virgin olive oil

2 cups sliced leeks, white and light green parts only, rinsed well or chopped onions

1½ cups diced carrots

1 tablespoon minced garlic (about 3 cloves)

1 (15½-ounce) can diced tomatoes

1 bay leaf

1 cup lentils, rinsed well and picked through for rocks

4 cups vegetable broth

½ teaspoon salt, or to taste

¼ teaspoon freshly ground black pepper, or to taste

Heat the olive oil in a large soup pot over medium-low heat. Sauté the leeks and carrots, stirring frequently, until the leeks wilt, about 5 minutes.

Stir in the garlic and immediately add the tomatoes, bay leaf, lentils, broth, salt, and pepper and bring to a boil over high heat. Reduce the heat and simmer, covered, until the lentils are the desired consistency, about 35–45 minutes (see note).

Remove the bay leaf and adjust salt if needed. Top with freshly ground black pepper, if desired. Serve by itself or over brown rice or quinoa.

Note: The cooking time will vary depending on the type of lentils you use. Brown lentils cook more quickly than French green lentils.

French Green Lentil Salad
with Asparagus and Pine Nuts

—JILL NUSSINOW—

I love the way that French green lentils hold their shape. You can use any nut in this dish, or none at all. The lemon zest has anticancer properties. Overall, this is a tasty dish for lunch, dinner or a special picnic.

Serves 4–6

1 cup chopped leek or onion

1½ cups French green lentils, rinsed

2½ cups water or stock (plus 1 for stove top cooking)

1½ cups thinly sliced asparagus

Juice and zest of 1 lemon or 2–3 tablespoons red wine or balsamic vinegar

Freshly ground black pepper, to taste

3 tablespoons toasted pine nuts

Salt, to taste (optional)

Chopped Italian parsley, for garnish

Dry sauté the leek over medium heat for 1 minute. Add 2½ cups and bring the mixture to a simmer over high heat. Reduce the heat and simmer, uncovered, adding water if necessary, until the lentils are cooked, about 25 minutes. (The lentils will still be firm but tender in the middle when thoroughly cooked).

Add the thinly sliced asparagus and simmer for 1–2 minutes until it is bright green.

Remove the mixture, using a slotted spoon to drain any excess liquid. Let the mixture cool by refrigerating or leaving at room temperature for 30 minutes.

Add the lemon zest and juice, ground black pepper and the pine nuts. Garnish with parsley.

M'jeddrah

—ELLEN KANNER—

A Middle Eastern dish both simple and elemental, the lentils and rice soak separately but cook together, taking on flavor and qualities greater than themselves. M'jeddrah is traditionally topped with a tumble of golden-brown sautéed onions. Paired with a salad or gorgeous green vegetable, it makes a meal.

Serves 4–6

1 cup brown lentils or French lentils, picked over and rinsed

1 cup brown rice

4 cups water or vegetable broth

1 bay leaf

2 tablespoons olive oil

1 large onion or two small, sliced thin

1 teaspoon cumin

Sea salt and fresh ground pepper to taste

Pour lentils into a small bowl. Cover with cold water. In a separate bowl, do the same with the rice. Leave 'em both to soak for 30 minutes or for up to 2 hours, if you've got the time. The lentils and rice don't need to be fussed with, just let them sit.

Bring water or vegetable broth to boil into a large saucepan. Strain lentils into a sieve. Rinse in cold water. Add to broth. Do the same with the brown rice. Toss in bay leaf. Bring to boil, reduce heat to low and cook, covered, for 30–40 minutes, until lentils and rice are gentled and fluffy and have soaked up all the liquid. Remove cover, remove from heat and set aside.

Just before serving, heat oil in a large skillet over medium-high heat. Add sliced onion and cook, stirring, for 3–5 minutes, until onions start to soften and turn golden and fragrant. Reduce heat to medium, and cook, stirring, another 10 minutes or so, until onions are burnished, glossy and tender. Season with sea salt and fresh ground pepper.

Stir lentils and rice together gently. Remove bay leaf, add cumin and season generously with sea salt and freshly ground pepper.

Top with all the golden onions and serve.

Nourishing Stew

—ELISA RODRIGUEZ—

This creamy comforting stew is a breeze to make! You can use canned and frozen ingredients for quick assembly in a crockpot or on your stovetop. This dish is free from gluten, corn, soy, grains, sulfites, yeast and nightshades, yet still has delicious flavor.

Serves 4–6

1 (24-ounce) can of chickpeas or 2½ cups cooked
1 (15-ounce) can of coconut milk
2 cups of quinoa, rinsed
1 head of organic Swiss chard, kale or collards, chopped coarsely
1 to 2 zucchini, diced
1 cup frozen peas
1 cup cauliflower, chopped
1 cup red lentils

2 leeks, sliced finely
¼ to ½ cup fresh squeezed lime juice
1 tablespoon cumin
1 teaspoon. turmeric
1 teaspoon ginger
1 teaspoon of Real, Himalayan or Sea salt (optional)
Fresh basil or parsley, chopped to garnish

Combine all ingredients (except fresh herbs) and cook gently on low until the flavors have melded together and the quinoa has expanded. I like to allow it to simmer most of the day for added flavor. Dish up, top with garnish, and enjoy this hearty stew knowing that you're nourishing your body.

Tips:

Use filtered water, as needed, to obtain desired consistency. This will vary based on the simmer time, amount of frozen veggies and canned liquids included. If the stew is more soup-like then stew-like, allow it to simmer longer and the excess liquid will evaporate.

You can prepare this recipe in a slow cooker, crock pot or on your stove top. Simply assemble and allow to simmer for several (4–6) hours. Make sure you have adequate liquid for longer cooking times. This dish tastes even better the next day, after the flavors have set.

There's no need to pre-cook the quinoa, it will absorb liquid and expand over time. I suggest checking back on the stew periodically and adding water as needed.

Red Lentil Soup
with Sweet Potatoes and Spinach

—ROBIN ASBELL—

Red lentils should be in every pantry, because they are so quick, delicious, and make a colorful soup! Add some sweet yams and a finishing touch of greens, and you have a satisfying meal. You can purée as instructed, for a thick and creamy soup, or simply eat as is, if you are in a hurry.

Serves 4–6

1 medium onion, chopped

1 medium carrot, chopped

2 cups sweet potato, cubed

1 cup red lentils, rinsed

1 tablespoon fresh rosemary, chopped

4 cups water

¼ cup white wine

5 ounces fresh spinach, 5 cups, packed

½ teaspoon salt

½ teaspoon cracked black pepper

In a soup pot, combine onion, carrot, sweet potato, red lentils, rosemary and water and bring to a boil. Reduce heat to low and cover tightly. Simmer for 30 minutes, checking and stirring halfway. When lentils are falling apart, stir in white wine and return to a simmer, then stir in the spinach, salt and pepper. Simmer just until the spinach is wilted, then take off the heat.

Scoop 3 cups of the soup into a food processor or blender and purée, then stir back into the pan. Serve hot.

Spicy Red Lentil Vegetable Soup

—JUDITH KINGSBURY—

For this lentil curry soup recipe, I use the small red lentils, known as Masoor Dahl, available in many natural food stores, or Indian groceries. They are light, easily digested, and cook very quickly. This red lentil soup recipe has many possible variations. The yam complements the red lentils very well, but add or substitute whatever vegetables you wish. Other kinds of lentils will work too, but they'll take longer to cook. I make this in the pressure cooker, but you make it in a pot on the stovetop, allowing it to cook for 25–35 minutes. This soup is good served with a scoop of rice, and a couple of Indian chapatis or tortillas, or any kind of sandwich. It's also good with orange raisin scones or oatmeal date nut muffins.

Serves 6

1 cup Indian red lentils
  (*Masoor Dahl*)

6 cups water

1 large yam (approximately
  1 pound), peeled and diced

1 cups sliced fresh green beans, cut
  into 1-inch sections

2 stalks celery, diced

½ red bell pepper, diced

1 teaspoon olive oil

2 thin slices fresh peeled ginger

1 cinnamon stick

1 bay leaf

1 pinch hing (asoefetida)

½ teaspoon ground fennel

½ teaspoon cumin seed

1 teaspoon ground coriander

½ teaspoon turmeric

½ teaspoon salt or to taste

2 tablespoons minced parsley, basil
  or cilantro as garnish

Clean, wash, rinse and drain the red lentils and add to pressure cooker. Add 6 cups water to lentils, bring to a boil, and skim the foam. Add the ginger slices, bay leaf, cinnamon stick. Lock on lid, bring to high pressure for 5 minutes, remove from heat, natural pressure release.

Prepare the veggies.

Heat the oil on medium in a large sauce pan and add the hing. Add the veggies, and sauté 5 minutes on med/high heat. Add the other spices, sauté briefly. Add 2 tablespoons water and stir to release the goodies on the bottom of the pan.

Stir the veggies and spices into the red lentils, lock on lid, bring back to high pressure for 2 minutes. Thin the soup with a little water or vegetable stock if it seems too thick. Stir in minced fresh herb, and serve with chapatis or rice.

To make on the stovetop: Cook the soup for about 30 minutes until the lentils are cooked through.

Rainbow Sprout Salad

—JILL NUSSINOW—

I recently ate something like this at a mushroom hunting potluck. I had already likely eaten too much but it was too beautiful and tasty to pass up. Vary the ingredients based on what you have available. Other great sprout additions are adzuki beans or whole green peas. (For more information on sprouting see the "Ingredient Sources" section on pages 244-245.)

Serves 4

1½ cups mung bean sprouts

1½ cups lentil sprouts

1 cup shredded red cabbage

½ cup shredded carrots

3 tablespoons toasted sunflower seeds

3 tablespoons dried cranberries or raisins (optional)

1 teaspoon grated orange zest

¼ cup freshly squeezed orange juice

2 tablespoons water

1–2 teaspoons mellow white miso

1–2 teaspoons Dijon mustard

1–2 teaspoons agave syrup (optional)

Combine all the vegetables in a bowl and toss, adding sunflower seeds and dried fruit, if using.

In a small bowl, combine orange juice, zest, water, miso, mustard and agave syrup, if using. Combine dressing with sprouts and vegetables right before serving. It can sit for up to 30 minutes, and it's even delicious as a leftover, if there is any, stuffed into tortillas, romaine or large collard leaves.

Minted Pea Soup

—JILL NUSSINOW—

This soup is refreshing and cooling, perfect for warmer weather. It only takes several minutes in the pressure cooker or 30 minutes on top of the stove.

Serves 4

1 tablespoon canola oil, optional

1½ cups chopped onions

1 cup diced new potatoes

1 cup peeled and chopped apples

3 cloves garlic, peeled and cut in half

2 bay leaves

½ teaspoon dried tarragon

½ teaspoon salt

3 cups water

2 cups fresh or frozen peas (reserving a few for garnish)

2 green leaf lettuce leaves

3 tablespoons chopped fresh Italian parsley

1 cup soy, or other non-dairy, milk

1–2 teaspoons fresh lemon juice, or to taste

2 tablespoons fresh chopped mint

Stovetop: Add the oil, if using, to a soup pot over medium heat. Sauté the onions for about 7 minutes, until translucent. Add the potatoes, apples, garlic, bay leaves, tarragon, salt and water and simmer for 20 minutes. Add the peas and place the lettuce leaves on top of peas. Simmer another 10 minutes. Remove the bay leaves. Add the parsley to the hot soup and purée with an immersion blender until smooth. Stir in the milk, lemon juice and chopped mint. Adjust seasonings, adding more salt, lemon juice or mint. Chill for at least 1 hour. Garnish with whole peas and serve.

Pressure Cooker: Sauté the onion for 5 minutes over medium heat. Add the potatoes, apples, garlic, bay leaves, tarragon, salt and water. Lock the lid on and bring to high pressure. Lower the heat to maintain high pressure for 3 minutes. Quick release the pressure. Add the peas and lettuce leaves. Return to high pressure for 2 minutes. Quick release the pressure.

Add the parsley and purée until smooth with an immersion blender. Stir in the milk, lemon juice and chopped mint. Adjust seasonings, adding more salt, lemon juice or mint. Chill for at least 1 hour. Garnish with whole peas and serve.

Thai Rice, Snow Pea and Mushroom Salad

—JILL NUSSINOW—

The flavors of Thai cooking are so enticing. Here they are combined to make an incredibly tasty salad. It is definitely rich since it uses coconut milk. I almost always use lite coconut milk since it adds the flavor with less fat. McDougallers must adjust this recipe. Omit the coconut milk and use 2¼ cups coconut or plain water to cook the rice. After it's cooked, stir in coconut extract for flavor. For the dressing use non-dairy milk, a pinch of guar or xanthan gum and coconut extract instead of coconut milk. Be sure to use all the seasonings, they are essential.

Serves 4–6

1½ cups brown jasmine or brown basmati rice, rinsed and soaked overnight, then drained

2 fresh stalks lemongrass, cut into 3 or 4 pieces

½ to 1 fresh chile, such as jalapeno or serrano, seeded and minced

1 teaspoon canola or other vegetable oil, optional

2 cups boiling water

¾ cup lite or regular coconut milk

½ teaspoon salt

DRESSING

¼ cup lite or regular coconut milk

3 tablespoons fresh lime juice

1 teaspoon sugar

½ teaspoon salt

2 tablespoons chopped fresh basil, preferably Thai basil

2 tablespoons chopped fresh cilantro or mint

1 medium red or orange pepper

½ pound snow peas, stemmed and cut in half diagonally

12 ounces assorted mushrooms, such as shiitake, crimini, oyster or white

2 teaspoons minced garlic

2 teaspoons grated fresh ginger root

1 whole kaffir lime leaf or if unavailable, 1 teaspoon lime zest and 2 teaspoons lime juice added at end of cooking

½ fresh chile, minced (seeded if you want it milder)

2 teaspoons canola or other vegetable oil, optional

Dash of salt

Chopped fresh Thai or regular basil

Roasted peanuts

In a small heavy pot with a tight fitting lid, sauté the rice, lemongrass and chile in the oil, if using, for 1–2 minutes, stirring constantly. Add the boiling water, coconut milk and salt and bring to a boil; then stir, reduce the heat to very low, cover and cook until all of the liquid has been absorbed, about 20 minutes.

Meanwhile, whisk together all of the dressing ingredients in a small bowl and set aside.

Seed the pepper and cut into thin strips about 1½ inches long. Blanch the pepper strips in boiling water for 1–2 minutes, until just tender, and set aside in a serving bowl. Blanch the snow peas in boiling water until just tender, about 1 minute and add to the serving bowl.

When the rice is tender, remove the lemongrass pieces, fluff the rice with a fork and set it aside to cool.

Remove and discard any tough stems from the mushrooms, then rinse and slice the caps into bite size pieces.

In a skillet, combine the garlic, ginger root, kaffir lime leaf, chile and oil, if using, and sauté on medium heat for 1 minute, stirring constantly. Add the mushrooms and salt and toss well. Cover the skillet, reduce the heat, and cook until the mushrooms are softened and begin to release their juices, about 3–5 minutes. Remove the lime leaf, then add the sautéed mushrooms and cooled rice to the serving bowl, pour on the dressing and toss well. Serve at room temperature, garnished with basil and peanuts.

Kale and Spring Pea Mash-up

—CARRIE FORREST—

This easy vegetable mix highlights kale and includes spring peas and a cooked sweet potato topped it with a satisfying Lemon-Tahini Sauce. You can use any type of kale for this recipe, but some say that lacinato (also known as "dino" or dinosaur kale) is less bitter than curly kale.

Serves 8

1 medium red onion, chopped

2 cups button mushrooms, sliced

2 tablespoons no-salt seasoning

1 tablespoon ground turmeric

1 medium tomato, chopped

1 (16-ounce) bag frozen spring peas, thawed

1 medium sweet potato, baked

1 cup black beans, rinsed and drained

1 (10-ounce) bag lacinato kale or two bunches, stems removed

¼ cup nutritional yeast

LEMON-TAHINI SAUCE

½ cup no-salt added jarred tahini

2 lemons

Defrost bag of peas overnight in refrigerator. Bake sweet potato. Wash and dry kale and remove stems. Chop onion and mushrooms. Drain and rinse beans.

Heat up a few tablespoons of water over medium heat in a large pot. Add onion and water-sauté for a few minutes or until soft. Add mushrooms and continue cooking for several more minutes.

Add no-salt seasoning and turmeric to the mixture and stir to combine. Add the tomato, peas, baked sweet potato and beans to the pot, along with about a ½ cup of water if mixture is dry. If using frozen peas, cook for longer. Stir to combine.

Finally, add the kale to the pot and turn the heat to low. Place the lid on the pot and cook for several minutes or until the kale is wilted but bright green. Turn the heat off and stir in the nutritional yeast and Lemon-Tahini Sauce.

For Lemon-Tahini Sauce: Place tahini in a medium bowl. Squeeze juice from lemons and add to tahini. Stir to blend. Use more or less lemon juice to reach desired flavor and consistency.

Creamy Southern Soup Beans

—NIKKI HANEY—

In the Appalachian Mountains, where I was born and raised, pinto beans have been a staple for generations. Our preferred serving style for these high fiber, low cholesterol legumes, is in a simple pot of Soup Beans. Traditionally, meat is added to the pot as the beans simmer to provide extra flavor. In this vegan version, the meat is removed and the soup's flavor comes from a combination of garlic, green onions and cashew cream. The Soup Beans thicken as they cool and some might argue that they taste better as leftovers than they do the first time around.

Serves 6

1 tablespoon whole raw cashews

2 cups dried pinto beans

1 garlic clove, peeled

sea salt, to taste

fresh ground black pepper, to taste

½ cup chopped green onions

Place the cashews in a small dish and add cold water until the cashews are fully submerged. Cover and refrigerate the cashews for 8–10 hours (or overnight). Drain the cashews and place them in a food processor along with enough cold water to just cover them. Blend until the cashews transform into a smooth cream.

Rinse the pinto beans and discard of any dark beans or rocky bits that you find while rinsing. Add the beans to a large pot and cover by 2-inches with water. Bring the beans to a boil, then reduce to a simmer. Add in the garlic clove and cover the pot. Cook the beans until tender, around 2 hours, stirring every 20 minutes and adding water as needed. When the beans are almost finished, add in the sea salt and pepper, to taste. Remove the beans from the heat. Stir in the chopped green onions and cashew cream. Cover the beans and allow the soup to thicken for at least 15 minutes before serving.

Store leftovers in an airtight container in the refrigerator for up to 3 days.

Pinto Bean Quinoa Burgers

—JILL NUSSINOW—

This will likely work with any cooked grain or bean with slight adjustments in amounts. I developed this recipe for one of the many Barbaras in my life who wanted something tasty and easy to eat.

Makes 6 medium

½ to ¾ cup cooked quinoa

1½ cups cooked pinto beans

¼ to ½ cup onion

2 cloves garlic

2 teaspoons ground cumin

Fresh herbs such as parsley, basil or cilantro

2 tablespoons nutritional yeast

½ teaspoon salt, if using fresh cooked, not canned, beans

2 tablespoons hemp seed, if you have it

Preheat oven to 350°F.

Put the quinoa, beans and onion in the food processor. Pulse a few times until slightly mixed. Add the garlic, cumin, herbs, yeast, and salt, if using. Pulse again, adding 1–2 tablespoons bean liquid, stock or *Bragg Liquid Aminos* if it needs it. Stir in hemp seeds. Form into patties. If the mixture doesn't feel thick enough, add more quinoa and combine again.

Bake on oiled baking sheet for 10 minutes. Turn over and bake another 10 minutes. Eat, refrigerate or freeze.

Miso Vegetable Soup

—JILL NUSSINOW—

While most people won't think of miso as a bean, it is most often made from fermented soy beans. I think that miso soup is a magical elixir. It is my go-to soup when my tummy is upset. I will usually eat a large bowl (or two) and it will get my digestive tract back on track. I have made it incredibly plain with just some wakame (seaweed) in it and a few slices of green onion, or I have added many more vegetables. Here I give you the vegetable variation.

Serves 2–4

1 piece wakame seaweed, soaked in hot water for at least 30 minutes

½ medium onion, sliced

1 medium carrot, thinly sliced on the diagonal

2 cups Napa (or other) cabbage or bok choy, sliced thin

1 cup broccoli florets or thin green beans

4 cups vegetable broth

¼ cup or more mellow white, or other, miso paste

2 tablespoons tamari, optional

2 green onions, sliced on the diagonal

Heat a saucepan over medium heat.

Remove the wakame from the water and cut out the center rib and cut the sides into small pieces.

Dry sauté the onion for 3–4 minutes. Add the carrot and 2 tablespoons of the broth and cook for 3 minutes. Add the cabbage or bok choy, 2 cups of the broth and the chopped wakame. Simmer for 2–3 more minutes and then add the broccoli and simmer another 2–3 minutes until the broccoli is almost cooked through. Remove ½ cup of the broth from the soup and add to a small bowl with the miso. Whisk to thoroughly combine and set aside.

Continue to cook the soup until all the vegetables are how you like them.

Remove the pot from the heat and add the tamari, if using, and the blended miso. Stir well. Ladle into bowls and garnish with the green onions.

Rice and Veggie Sushi Salad

—JILL NUSSINOW—

Inspired by a recipe in Moosewood Restaurant Lowfat Favorites, *this recipe was one of the winners in "John Ash's Good Food Hour" rice recipe contest sponsored by KSRO, my local radio station. John said that he loved the clean flavors. I like it because it tastes like sushi, only better, since I can add many vegetables. I use brown, not sushi, rice because I like the texture better. This contains not only edamame, green soybeans, but mung bean sprouts for a double dose of legumes.*

Serves 4–6

1 cup short grain brown rice
1½ cups water
¼ cup rice vinegar
2 tablespoons ume plum vinegar
2 tablespoons *Sucanat* or sugar
2 teaspoons grated fresh ginger
1 teaspoon wasabi powder and
  1 teaspoon water
2 medium carrots, peeled and diced
1 cup fresh or frozen, thawed green
  soybeans, also called edamame

½ cup diced daikon radish
1 cup mung bean sprouts
¼ cup sliced green onions
1 ripe avocado, cut into chunks
1 sheet toasted nori seaweed
2 tablespoons black or brown sesame
  seeds, toasted
Washed Asian greens, like mizuna,
  tatsoi or red mustard

Bring the water to a boil in a medium saucepan. Stir in the rice. Cover and reduce the heat to a simmer. Cook for 40 minutes, then remove from the heat and let stand for 10 minutes (or pressure cook for 20 minutes with a natural pressure release.)

While the rice is cooking blanch the carrots and edamame in boiling water or steam for 2–3 minutes.

In a non-reactive bowl, such as glass or stainless steel, combine the rice vinegar, ume vinegar, *Sucanat,* ginger and wasabi.

Tear the nori sheet into small strips and combine with the sesame seeds. In a large bowl, combine the cooked warm rice with the vinegar sauce and the vegetables, except the avocado.

To Serve: Carefully combine the avocado. Sprinkle the rice mixture with the nori-sesame mixture. Put the greens on plates and serve the rice salad on top.

Note: When other vegetables are in season, such as cucumber, red pepper, peas or summer squash, use them in this salad. Also, you can mix in any leftover cooked vegetables such as green beans or broccoli florets.

Chef AJ's 8 Minute Split Pea Soup

—CHEF AJ—

Making soup doesn't get easier than this. You can substitute yellow split peas for the green ones and sweet potatoes for the white potatoes. You can also cook this in a pot on the stove and it will take 30–45 minutes for the split peas to cook through.

Serves 6–8

- 1 pound of green split peas
- 1 large chopped onion (I use the 10-ounce bag, precut from *Trader Joe's*)
- 1 pound carrots, sliced
- 1 bunch celery, sliced (you can actually buy mirepoix, celery, carrots and onions already chopped at *Trader Joe's*)
- 2 large Russet potatoes, cubed
- 8 cups boiling water
- 6–8 cloves garlic, pressed
- 4 teaspoons chopped parsley, dried (not fresh)
- 1–2 tablespoons salt-free seasoning*
- 1 teaspoon basil
- 1 teaspoon rosemary
- 1 teaspoon oregano
- 1 teaspoon celery seed
- 1 teaspoon smoked paprika
- 1 bay leaf
- 1 capful *Wright's Liquid Smoke,* optional

Place all ingredients in an electric pressure cooker. Cook on high for 8 minutes. Let pressure release naturally. Stir in one capful of *Wright's Liquid Smoke*, if desired.

Tastes even better the next day!

---

*My favorite is *Benson's Table Tasty* which is available online.

The Pressure Cooker and Pulses Can Save Your Life or at Least Your Time

Pulses? In case you were randomly flipping through this book and didn't already read it, pulses are dried beans, peas and lentils. Generally they take a long time to cook, even the lentils and peas which don't need to be presoaked take a longer time to cook than most people want to spend. This is where the pressure cooker performs its magic on pulses.

You can cook beans from dry to cooked or from soaked to cooked. I prefer the latter method as I find that soaking improves the chances that all my beans will be cooked through. I also use far less energy when I've used soaked beans as it requires little effort to put beans in a bowl or glass jar and add water, and let them sit, overnight or from the morning until the evening.

Once soaked, the beans are drained and then added to the pressure cooker. Soaked beans such as black, navy, kidney and pinto take just 6 minutes at pressure. Chickpeas take 12–14 minutes at pressure. This is fast. You can barely get into your car and drive to the store, grab a can of beans, and get back home before your pressure cooker beans will be finished cooking.

Many people love the electric pressure cooker but my first love has been the stove top model. The benefit of the electric pressure cooker is that you can set it and then walk away and it automatically goes to the warm setting. You don't have to be home to get your beans, soup or chili recipe completed.

To give you brief advice on pressure cooking pulses, use 1 cup dry beans to 2 cups water and cook for 20–25 minutes for standard beans. If the beans are soaked, use ½ to ¾ cup water per cup of soaked dry beans. Cook for 6 minutes at pressure. For lentils and split peas, use the 1:2 ratio but cook at pressure for 6 minutes. Let the pressure come down naturally with beans for the best results.

When you cook pulses, make extra and freeze them to use later. If you can, and want to, freeze the beans on a cookie sheet and then freeze in bags or jars. You will be able to take out as many beans as you want. If not, then freeze in one and ½ cup amounts which is what you will find in a 15 ounce can of beans. You will soon see that you can say goodbye to those cans of beans, except for emergencies.

—Jill Nussinow

Split Pea and Yam Soup

—CATHY FISHER—

Sweet yams and earthy greens add a new level of excitement to traditional split pea soup. This recipe is very easy to make and yields a large pot of soup, perfect for a family dinner or lunches for the week.

Serves 6

9 cups water

2 cups dry split peas

1 medium yellow onion, chopped

1 medium yam, peeled and diced

1 medium white potato, peeled and diced

2 ribs celery, chopped

1 teaspoon granulated garlic

1 teaspoon dried oregano

½ teaspoon ground cumin

¼ teaspoon ground celery seed

½ to 1 bunch greens (kale, chard, collards), chopped into bite-size pieces

Fill a large soup pot with the water and split peas and bring to a boil. Turn down to a low-medium boil (not a simmer) and cook for 30 minutes, stirring occasionally.

Add the onion, yam, potato, celery, garlic, oregano, cumin, and celery seed, and continue to cook, now at a medium boil, for about 20 minutes until the potatoes are soft, stirring occasionally. Add a little water as needed.

Add in the greens and cook for an additional 10 minutes. Serve hot.

Optional: Garnish with chopped tomatoes, sliced celery or fresh oregano.

Note about soup texture: Create a smoother soup by using a handheld potato masher or electric immersion blender, or by pouring half or all of the soup into a blender or food processor (cool a bit first before doing this so there is no danger of burning yourself).

Asian Bean Dip

—JILL NUSSINOW—

This tantalizing dip was created in front of a McDougall cooking class, on the fly. Luckily, someone wrote down the ingredients. It was their favorite dip of the day. You'll notice that the beans aren't Asian but I suspect that it would also work well with cooked adzuki, mung or soybeans.

Makes about 2 cups

1 clove garlic

1–2 tablespoons peanut butter

1 1-inch piece of ginger, peeled

1½ cups cooked cannellini beans

1 teaspoon rice vinegar

1 tablespoon mellow white, or any other, miso

3 tablespoons water

1 tablespoon or more cilantro leaves

1 tablespoon sugar, *Sucanat* or equivalent sugar substitute

1 green onion, sliced

Put the garlic, peanut butter and ginger in a food processer and process until finely chopped. Add the beans, vinegar, miso and water and blend until slightly chunky. Add the cilantro, sweetener and green onion and process briefly until combined. Taste and adjust the seasonings to your liking by adding more vinegar, miso or sugar.

Use as a dip for vegetables or rice crackers or as a filling for wraps.

Pasta with Zesty Lemon White Bean Sauce

—TESS CHALLIS—

This hearty, zippy pasta dish is sure to satisfy! This recipe makes a very generous amount of sauce, which is how it's traditionally served—a nice big portion of bean sauce over a light portion of pasta. However, feel free to customize the proportions so that it's just right for you!

Serves 4

8 ounces whole grain pasta

2 (15-ounce) cans white beans or 3 cups beans (cannellini, northern beans, etc.), drained and rinsed

10 large cloves garlic, minced or pressed

½ cup plain, unsweetened non-dairy milk

¼ cup fresh lemon juice

1 tablespoon minced lemon zest (the zest of 2 medium-large lemons)

4 teaspoons extra-virgin olive oil

1 teaspoon sea salt

½ teaspoon black pepper

2 tablespoons (packed) fresh basil, cut into thin ribbons

Cook the pasta al dente according to the directions on the package. Drain and set aside. You'll be able to make the rest of the dish in the time the pasta cooks.

Place the drained beans in a medium pot and smash them, using a potato masher. Leave in plenty of texture, but smash them until they've gotten a bit creamy. Add the remaining sauce ingredients and stir well. Heat over medium until thoroughly warmed, about 5 minutes, stirring often. Remove from heat and set aside.

Serve the pasta topped with generous portions of the sauce and sprinkled with the basil.

Tuscan Soup with a Twist

—ELLEN JONES—

Even in Florida, it gets bone-chilling cold in the winter. This soup will satisfy the core of your comfort food cravings, but warm and protect you against the worst of winter's fury. In my opinion, you can never have too many allium family/cancer-fighting onions. Feel free to add or subtract according to your tastes. The light-colored beans give this soup its creamy consistency.

Serves 4–6 (or just you 4 to 6 times)

2 cups vegetable broth plus
4 tablespoons for sautéing

1 cup cooked garbanzo beans

1 cup cooked cannellini or
white beans

8 ounces button mushrooms,
chopped

1 yellow onion, chopped

1 bunch, green onions, thinly sliced
plus 1 tablespoon for garnish

2 tablespoons chopped flat parsley
plus 1 tablespoon for garnish

2 tablespoons chopped chives

½ teaspoon salt (optional)

Freshly ground black pepper (optional)

In a blender, add the vegetable broth, garbanzo beans and cannellini beans. Process until all of the beans are blended into a creamy consistency. Add more water, a tablespoon at a time to achieve a creamier consistency if desired.

In a large soup pot add the mushrooms and onions. Add two tablespoons of the vegetable broth and sauté over medium heat until the vegetables are translucent. Add a tablespoon of broth at a time to keep the vegetables from sticking. Add the bean mixture and parsley, and stir well over low heat until the soup is steaming hot.

Serve into bowls and garnish with the parsley and chives. Add salt and pepper to taste.

Slow Cooker Yellow-Eyed Bean Soup
with Sweet Potatoes and Greens

—KATHY HESTER—

I fell in love with yellow eyed beans the first time I tasted them last year. Prettier than black-eyed peas they have a smoother texture too. They were traditionally used in baked beans but are also great in Southern faves, soups and stews. In this soup the sweet potatoes mix with the beans to create a rich broth with a hint of sweetness. Don't have yellow eyed beans? Use black-eyed peas, pintos or another heirloom bean you've been saving.

Serves 4–6

2 cup sweet potato, diced

2 cup dried yellow eyed beans

4 cloves garlic, minced

6 cups water

2 tablespoon veggie bouillon

2 (2-inch) sprig fresh rosemary or ¾ teaspoon ground

3 teaspoon marjoram

1 teaspoon smoked paprika

4 cups chopped greens (collards, kale, spinach, etc.)

2–3 tablespoons nutritional yeast (leave out if your bouillon has yeast in it already)

a few drops liquid smoke, optional

a few drops garlic *Tabasco,* optional

salt and pepper, to taste

Add the sweet potato, beans, garlic, water, bouillon, rosemary, marjoram and paprika into your 3½ to 5 quart slow cooker. Cook on low 8–10 hours.

Fifteen minutes before serving add the greens. Also add the nutritional yeast, liquid smoke and *Tabasco* if you are using it. You can also add more water if you'd prefer it thinner.

Right before serving add salt and pepper, taste, then adjust any of the seasonings as needed.

C H A M P S

Seeds and Nuts Included

Almonds

Brazil Nuts

Cashews

Chia Seeds

Flax Seeds

Hemp Seeds

Macadamia Nuts

Peanuts

Pumpkin Seeds

Sesame Seeds

Sunflower Seeds

Walnuts

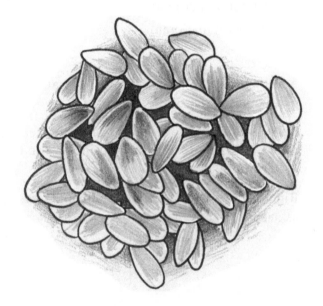

CHAPTER 6

Seeds and Nuts

D O Y O U K N O W the joke about people who live in California? It's where all the nuts and fruits go to live. Well, what about those of us who are seedy? I think that we are here, too.

One of my sayings is, I am nuts about nuts. And it's true. While some people eschew nuts because they are high in fat, I like to eat them often in small amounts. I think that they make plant-based food more palatable. They are meant to be condiments and small additions, not the basis for your meal.

Many people have gone cashew-crazy lately, adding them to many dishes in the form of a thickener. I have some recipes for cashew crème but I don't eat it every day or even every week. I love almond butter but I don't eat that everyday either. Soaked almonds are part of my husband's morning green smoothie. When it comes to nuts, err on the side of eating less rather than eating more unless you need to pack on the pounds. (If that's you, we need to talk…)

If you think about the way that natural nuts come from the trees (or bushes if they are peanuts which are truly legumes or pulses), they are in shells. Yet modern technological advances have made shelled nuts much more available than those in their shells. Did you ever notice how hard the squirrels and crows need to work to get the nuts out of their shells? If you have, that's what we need to be doing. I can assure you that you will be eating far fewer nuts if you arm yourself with a nutcracker and nuts-in-the-shell than if you have a bowl or (goodness forbid) a can of nuts at your disposal. Think of using small amounts when it comes to nuts and the goodness that they can add to your food.

A study in the *New England Journal of Medicine* from November 2013 stated that: "Increased nut consumption has been associated with a reduced risk of major chronic diseases, including cardiovascular disease and type 2 diabetes mellitus." Those who were most positively affected consumed nuts seven or more times per week. Previous studies have shown increased nut consumption associated with reduced waist circumference, less weight gain, and a decreased risk of obesity. Nuts tend to make you feel more satiated. Portion size makes a difference, as I previously stated.

For many people seeds are a better choice than nuts because they are not quite as fatty, are higher in protein, and a bit less tantalizing, although I think that they are mighty delicious. Some seeds are easy to eat such as sunflower and pumpkin because they are large enough to get a grip on. Less easy to consume, but equally as important, are sesame, hemp, flax and chia seeds because they are so small. I rarely eat poppy seeds because they manage to lodge in the crevices in my teeth and I don't care for that.

A few sesame seeds sprinkled here or there on top of dishes works well. Hemp seeds make their way to my nightly salads. Flax must be ground in order to be absorbed, and then it makes a wonderful topping on oats, or a binder in burgers and baking. Chia can be soaked and made into a gel or ground and used as a binder, too.

Flax, hemp and chia are amazing sources of essential Omega-3 fatty acids which help keep your immune system in order and keep your system moving. Flax is also beneficial in protecting against heart disease because it contains lignans, a type of fiber.

All nuts and seeds contain important fiber, protein and fat, in its natural form. Each nut or seed brings something to the party. Flax and sesame have anti-cancer properties. (Don't be surprised if in the future we find out more amazing properties of seeds and nuts.)

Sesame seeds are a rich source of calcium. They also contain Vitamin E. While I enjoy my sesame seeds, whole raw and toasted, my favorite way to eat them is as tahini. I eat a teaspoon of tahini most days, on my food or in my food as part of a simple sauce mixed with miso, lemon or lime juice and sometimes with garlic.

The potential benefits of eating sesame seeds include blood sugar and blood pressure regulation, reducing inflammation, and mood boosting. I know that when I eat sesame seeds I often feel better but this is, of course, anecdotal.

Pumpkin seeds which are rich in iron and calcium and are a good source of zinc which is essential for good immune health.

Feeling Nutty?

Like all other plant foods nuts are a source of antioxidants, vitamins and minerals plus protein and fat, mostly, with some carbohydrates. It's best to buy raw nuts whenever possible. Store them in the refrigerator or freezer to keep them fresh. (Not all the nuts listed here are included in the recipes but you can often substitute one nut for another, unless you are talking about me.)

Almonds are rich in fiber and Vitamin E. They might also help lower cholesterol and help stabilize blood sugar. They are one of the nuts lowest in fat.

1 ounce = 23 nuts, 160 calories and contains 14 grams fat.

Brazil nuts are perhaps the homeliest of the nuts but just 1 of them supplies more than 100 percent of the daily value of selenium which might help prevent bone, prostate and breast cancer. Consuming too much selenium can be harmful so eat them less often and eat just one or two.

1 ounce = 5–6 nuts, 185 calories and contains 18 grams of fat.

Cashews are a good source of iron, zinc and magnesium, a mineral also found in dark green leafy vegetables. Magnesium might help protect against age-related memory loss.

1 ounce = 18 nuts, 165 calories and contains 13 grams fat.

Hazelnuts/Filberts contain high levels of monounsaturated fats which can improve cardiovascular health. They also can help regulate blood sugar which is important for type 2 diabetics.

21 nuts = 180 calories and contains 17 grams of fat.

Macadamia are the nut that is the highest in monounsaturated fats which can be heart-healthy although they are one of the most calorie-dense nuts so it might be easy to eat too many. They might help lower cholesterol and triglycerides.

1 ounce = 10 nuts, 200 calories and contains 22 grams of fat.

Peanuts are technically legumes but generally referred to as nuts. They are high in folate — a mineral essential for brain development that may protect against cognitive decline. Like most other nuts, peanuts are also full of brain-boosting healthy fats and Vitamin E. They also contain resveratrol which is the antioxidant component of red wine that makes it so beneficial.

1 ounce = about 28 unshelled nuts, 170 calories and contains 14 grams of fat.

Pecans may help improve heart health by lowering cholesterol and might be brain protective. They can be used instead of walnuts in many recipes.

1 ounce = about 18 halves, 200 calories and contains 21 grams of fat.

Pine nuts or *pignoli* are tasty little treats. In the past few years their price has gone up dramatically and often the ones imported from China cause some people to get "pine nut mouth" which causes everything to taste like metal. Pay attention to the place of origin. These nuts help quell hunger and you don't need to add many to add a bit of richness to a recipe. They are the nut traditionally used to make pesto.

1 ounce = about 150 nuts, 188 calories, contains 19 grams of fat.

Pistachios are the slimmest nut with only 4 calories per nut. If you buy them in the shell that ought to slow down your consumption of this tasty nut. It might be best to count them out and put the bag away. Pistachios may reduce lung cancer risk.

1 ounce = 40 nuts, 160 calories, contains 14 grams of fat.

Walnuts are the nut richest in Omega-3 fatty acids, which help boost your immune system and fight inflammation. They are a good source of the mineral manganese.

1 ounce = 14 walnut halves, 185 calories, contains 18 grams of fat.

Nut and seed butters contain the same things as the nuts and seeds from which they are derived but they are much easier to eat and it's more difficult to monitor your consumption, especially if you don't use level measuring tablespoons. What some people think is a tablespoon of nut butter is probably two tablespoons. So use them with caution.

Nuts and seeds are condiments and do not make the whole meal. Enjoy their richness but in small, tasty doses. If nuts and seeds are a "problem food" for you, ban them from your household and your possession. You can live a "just fine," and maybe better, life without them. You know who you are.

Kale Apple Almond Milk

—RITA RIVERA—

For a change of pace make this sweet green milk.

Makes 16 ounces

1½ cups apple juice

½ cup filtered water

1 cup almonds

1 cup kale, stemmed and coarsely chopped

Preparing the kale: Remove the stems and coarsely chop the kale. Gently press the kale down into the measuring cup for measurement.

Preparing the almonds: I suggest you soak the almonds overnight, approximately 8–10 hours. Rinse them well and proceed with the recipe.

Add all ingredients to blender. Blend well. Strain through a cheese cloth or nut milk bag. Drink immediately or refrigerate.

Raw Almond Matcha Cakes

—ERIN WYSOCARSKI—

This is a great way to use up the pulp that's left over after making homemade almond milk. These little cakes are rich and sweet — and look brilliantly green and adorable once formed.

Makes 12–14 cakes

2 cups raw almond pulp

¼ cup raw agave syrup

½ tablespoons matcha (green tea) powder

1½ teaspoons wheatgrass powder

1 tablespoon raw virgin coconut oil (at room temperature)

¼ cup tahini

⅛ teaspoon salt (or more to taste)

Combine all of the ingredients in a large bowl. Using your hands, incorporate well and shape using cookie cutters or form into balls. Refrigerate between waxed paper for about an hour to set.

Red Almond Cheese

—SHARON GREENSPAN—

This colorful cheese will bring "oohs" and "ahs" to your table! Serve on cucumber rounds topped with a piece of red pepper or as a sauce over your favorite vegetables or pasta. Almonds are a heart healthy food and help to regulate cholesterol.

When made as directed, this cheese will ferment, slightly, forming valuable probiotics. If you prefer to make it for immediate consumption, use ¼ cup water instead of 1½ cups and reduce the salt by half.

Serves 4–6

1½ cups organic raw almonds

Ample water for soaking nuts

1½ cups chopped organic red pepper

3 tablespoons organic lime juice

½ teaspoon salt (sea, Celtic or Himalayan)

1½ cups clean water

Put the nuts in a jar and soak overnight (or all day). You will not see tails.

Pour the water out through a strainer, discarding the soaking water.

Put all ingredients and clean water in a blender. Blend on low or pulse a few times, and then blend on high until it becomes paste.

Put into a jar and cover with cheesecloth. There will be expansion as the cheese ferments, so be sure to leave an extra inch of head room. You may want to sprinkle a little salt on top. Allow to sit at room temperature overnight (or all day). Liquid will sink to the bottom and the cheese will rise to the top.

Remove cheesecloth and eat! Spoon the cheese out of the jar. You may ingest or discard the liquid. Store leftovers tightly covered for 3–5 days in the refrigerator. The taste will change and you can keep it for about a week to 10 days.

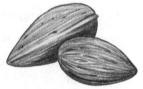

Romaine Burritos

—KAREN RANZI—

This is a simple light lunch or dinner. The filling will keep for a few days but won't likely last that long.

Serves 4–6

One bunch large Romaine lettuce leaves

TACO FILLING

1 cup almonds or walnuts, soaked 8–12 hours

½ cup lemon juice

¼ cup sun-dried tomatoes, soaked 2 hours, chopped

2 tablespoons chopped red onion

1 teaspoon each ground cumin, coriander and paprika (can substitute ¼ cup fresh cilantro for the ground coriander)

Put all ingredients into a food processor with an S-blade. Process until smooth, or until the consistency of a traditional bean dip. Add a little water if needed to get moving. Add fresh tomato salsa on top for an extra taste treat. Put a few tablespoons of the filling inside a Romaine lettuce leaf, roll up and eat.

Umami Sun-Dried Tomato and Almond Burgers

—DREENA BURTON—

These have fast become one of my FAVE burger recipes! The flavor is full of umami depth from the nuts, tamari, and sun-dried tomatoes. They taste fantastic paired with sliced avocado in burger buns or wrapped in whole-grain tortillas!

Serves 6

2 cups raw almonds

1 small to medium clove garlic, cut in quarters

2 tablespoons balsamic vinegar

1 tablespoon tamari (or liquid coconut amino acids)

1½ tablespoons tomato paste

¼ teaspoon sea salt

½ teaspoon dried rosemary (or 1½ teaspoon fresh rosemary leaves)

¾ to 1 cup green onions, sliced

½ cup sun-dried tomatoes (not oil-packed; preferably pre-sliced or chop before adding to processor, see note)

1½ cups cooked quinoa (cooled first; can substitute brown rice)

In a food processor, add almonds, garlic, balsamic, tamari, tomato paste, rosemary, and salt. Purée until the nuts are very finely ground, and becoming a little sticky. Be sure to grind them fine enough so that the almonds release some oils and become a little 'sticky', which will help bind the burgers — you don't want almond butter, but a very fine meal that is becoming clumpy.

Then add green onions and sun-dried tomatoes and pulse through until the mixture becomes dense and is starting to hold together. Add quinoa and process/pulse through again until well incorporated.

Remove blade, and shape into patties (or refrigerate first for ½ hour, which makes it easier to shape patties).

To cook, heat a non-stick skillet over medium heat. Cook patties, about 5–7 minutes on first side, and then another 3–5 minutes on second side until golden brown. These patties hold their shape well, but if they are flipped a lot and overcooked they become more crumbly and dry. Serve with fixings of choice.

Sun-dried tomato note: Some varieties/brands of sun-dried tomatoes can be very tough and hard, and others quite soft. If the ones you have are soft, go ahead and add them straight — but if they are very hard, it is useful to soak them in boiling water for a few minutes to soften (fully drain and pat dry before adding to processor).

High-Fiber Blueberry, Pear, and Spinach Smoothie
with Brazil Nuts

—JOANNE WILLIAMS—

Brazil nuts are a great addition to any smoothie. They are the most concentrated food source of selenium, an important trace mineral that acts as an antioxidant against free radicals. A single nut meets your daily requirement.

Requires a High-Speed Blender

Makes 4 (1-cup) servings

1½ cups room-temperature water

4 raw Brazil nuts (soaking not necessary)

1 (1-gram) packet stevia powder (optional)

2 cups organic baby spinach

2 ripe medium organic pears, cored and cut into 8 pieces

1½ cups frozen blueberries

2 teaspoons cold-pressed flax seed oil

Place the water, Brazil nuts, and stevia in a blender and blend until smooth and milky.

Add the spinach, pears, and blueberries, with the blueberries on top, and blend until smooth.

Add the flax seed oil, blend briefly, and serve immediately.

Creamy Cashew Almond Custard

—RITA RIVERA—

Use the "Cashew Almond Date Milk" on page 205 — made without the dates — to make this tasty dessert.

Makes 4 half cup servings

2 cups cashew almond milk
  (see note above)

1 cup coconut palm sugar

1½ teaspoons powdered (not flake) agar agar

1 teaspoon of ground vanilla beans, or ½ teaspoon vanilla extract

Place milk and powdered agar agar in saucepan and heat on medium, continually whisking. Once the mixture has warmed add the coconut palm sugar, again continually whisking.

Continue to whisk the mixture. Just before boiling, remove from stove and add the vanilla. Do not let the mixture boil.

Pour into a dish and let cool for a few hours. Once it has cooled place in the refrigerator for another 2–3 hours. The mixture should be solid. Break into pieces and place in blender. Blend well but do not add any additional liquid. If necessary, stop and start the blender until the mixture blends into a creamy texture.

Pour into serving cups. Garnish with powdered cinnamon, or chocolate sauce.

Notes:

Why soak your nuts? A soak stimulates the germination process and any enzyme inhibitors will be released into the soak water, which should then be discarded.

What are enzyme inhibitors? These special enzymes keep a seed or nut in a "dormant" state until conditions are right for sprouting. By neutralizing the enzyme inhibitors, the germination growth stage is stimulated, activiting the beneficial enzymes. These beneficial enzymes assist in the digestibility of nutrients.

Cashew Almond Date Milk

—RITA RIVERA—

Use this fresh "milk" instead of what comes in a box or carton. You will find it amazingly refreshing.

Makes 16 ounces

2 cups filtered water

½ cup cashews

¼ cup almonds

2 medjool dates, medium/large, pitted

Soak the almonds overnight, approximately 8–10 hours. Soak the cashews approximately 4 hours. Rinse them well and proceed with the recipe.

Blend all ingredients well. Strain through a cheese cloth or nut milk bag. Drink immediately or refrigerate.

Creamy House Dressing

—DREENA BURTON—

This thick, creamy dressing has no added oil, and has the greatest umami taste with the combination of seasonings. It's quick, easy, and might just become your new staple sauce!

Serves 4–8

½ cup soaked cashews (see note)

⅓ cup water

1 tablespoon tahini

1 tablespoon tamari or coconut amino acids

1½ to 2 tablespoon red wine vinegar (adjust to taste)

2 to 2½ teaspoons pure maple syrup (adjust to taste)

1½ teaspoons Dijon mustard

⅛ teaspoon salt

Freshly ground black pepper to taste

1 tablespoon sliced green onions

Optional: 1 teaspoon fresh chopped thyme, or ½ teaspoon fresh chopped rosemary

In a blender or with a immersion blender and deep cup, add all ingredients (starting with 1½ tablespoons vinegar and 2 teaspoons maple syrup) and process until smooth and creamy. If using a high-powered blender, this will smooth out very quickly. If using a standard blender/immersion blender, it will take a few minutes of blending. Once smooth, taste, and add additional vinegar/syrup to taste.

Cashews Note: Raw cashews take about 3–4 hours to soak, so I find it helpful to soak in batches and then freeze in portions until ready to use. To soak, place nuts in a bowl of water and cover for several hours. The nuts will become larger after soaking, as they swell from absorbing some of the water. Drain the soaking water, and rinse the nuts. Then store in the fridge for a couple of days until ready to use, or in the freezer for a few months.

Raw Cashew and Tahini Dressing

—ERIN WYSOCARSKI—

Rich and creamy, with a slight tang, this five-ingredient dressing is a perfect complement to a raw kale salad. It's easy to whip up, and addictive after the first bite. This may also be tossed with raw kale and dehydrated to make kale chips.

Serves 4–6

¾ cup raw cashews (dry or soaked overnight)

¾ cup raw tahini

2 teaspoons raw apple cider vinegar

1 cup water

¼ teaspoon salt

Grind the cashews in a small food processor until very crumbly, about a minute. Add in the rest of the ingredients and process until smooth, about a minute more.

To make the salad, place washed and dried kale pieces into a large prep bowl. Douse the kale with some of the dressing, then stir it around in the bowl in a circular motion. Serve immediately.

This also makes a great coating for kale chips. Place the coated kale into a food dehydrator set at 130°F for 8 hours.

Store leftover dressing in a glass container. It may be kept in the refrigerator for up to a week.

Wonder Spread

—DREENA BURTON—

This recipe has such simple ingredients, that you might think it doesn't taste particularly special. But it does! Spread on breads, use for sandwiches, wraps, baked potatoes, veggie burgers, or mix into grains or vegetable dishes. Be forewarned, this spread (or dip, sauce, mayo!) is addictive!

Makes about 1½ cups

- 1 cup soaked cashews (soak in advance, see note)
- 1½ tablespoons chickpea miso (see note)
- 2 tablespoons nutritional yeast
- 1½ tablespoons freshly squeezed lemon juice
- ¼ teaspoon pure maple syrup
- ½ cup water
- Salt and pepper if desired, to taste

In a blender, purée all ingredients on high speed until very smooth. Season to taste with additional salt if desired. Spread on breads, use for sandwiches, wraps, baked potatoes, veggie burgers, or to mix into grains or vegetable dishes. Many serving options with this recipe, it is delicious! Transfer to airtight containers to refrigerate.

Miso Note: Chickpea miso is something I discovered this past year. It has such a mild, mellow flavor and a very fermented, umami essence. If you cannot find it, use a very mild miso like a brown rice — and start with just 1 tablespoon as it tastes stronger than chickpea miso.

Crazy for Coconut

I am not really sure what turned the tides about coconut as part of our food supply but these days if you aren't eating it or wearing it, you just aren't with it.

When I went to school to become a dietitian they told us that coconut oil is the most saturated fat and that it's not good for you. At the same time they mentioned that it contains medium-chain triglycerides which won't raise your cholesterol. So there are a couple of opposing factors here. And, for about 25 years this didn't matter at all.

Then the coconut craze started and people were asking if coconut oil is OK. Beyond that, we now have coconut butter, which contains some of the coconut meat, coconut milk which is the creamy part of the coconut, often blended up, sometimes with sugar added, and coconut water which can be unsweetened or also have sugar added. Then there is "lite" coconut milk which appears to be regular coconut milk with extra water.

For the big question, is coconut oil OK to use? Drum roll, please...

The answer depends upon whether or not you use any added oil and how you feel about added fat. I think that most people who follow a raw food diet are probably consuming too much coconut. It makes sense to me that if you live in a tropical climate or have that in your family history or genetics perhaps you can eat plenty of coconut, but for the rest of us, we don't need much coconut to get our fat. We will likely do just fine with the more temperate fats such as the ones contained in nuts, seeds, olives and avocados.

If you use coconut water or even some coconut milk once in a while, it's not likely going to be the big thing that kills you or makes you sick. That's why I decided to include this recipe for Dr. Shiroko Sokitch's Favorite Breakfast. Sokitch is a medical doctor who has a holistic practice, incorporating acupuncture and Chinese medicine in Santa Rosa, CA where I live. She says that this recipe fills her up and is very satisfying. Sometimes she stirs cooked oats into it, as well.

1 cup of organic coconut milk

2 tablespoons chia seeds

1 tablespoon hemp seeds

1 tablespoon almond butter

Drizzle of pomegranate syrup or dried fruit or sweetener

Boil the coconut milk, then stir in the seeds and let sit for 5 minutes until the chia seeds plump up. Put into a bowl and stir in the almond butter. Drizzle with pomegranate syrup.

—Jill Nussinow

Banana Nut Chia Pudding

—KATJA HEINO—

Chia seeds are an amazing superfood loaded with fiber, protein, and antioxidants. They are also an excellent source of Omega-3 oils. Two tablespoons of chia seeds contain 7 grams of fiber, 2 grams of protein, and 5 grams of Omega-3. Prepare this pudding the night before, and you will have an instant, nutritious breakfast in the morning. Ridiculously easy to make and keeps you full for hours. This recipe easily doubles to serve 4–6 people.

Serves 2–3

- 2 cup homemade coconut or nut milk (or store bought)
- 2 bananas
- 4 dates, pitted (or 2 tablespoons pure maple syrup)
- 1 teaspoon vanilla extract
- Pinch of cinnamon
- 4 tablespoons chia seeds

TOPPINGS

- ¼ cup raisins
- 2 tablespoons raw cashews, roughly chopped
- 2 tablespoons raw almonds, roughly chopped

Place all topping ingredients into glass jar and cover with filtered water. Place in fridge or set on counter to soak overnight.

Place milk, dates (or maple syrup), bananas, cinnamon, and vanilla, into high powered blender. Process until smooth and dates are all broken up and incorporated.

Pour into glass jar. Add chia seeds and cover with tight fitting lid. Shake until well incorporated.

Let sit in fridge overnight (or at least 4 hours).

In the morning, drain the toppings and rinse well. Pour over chia pudding.

Overnight Muesli

—CHEF AJ—

Muesli was introduced around 1900 by the Swiss physician Maximilian Bircher-Benner for patients in his hospital, where a diet rich in fresh fruit and vegetables was an essential part of therapy. Muesli in its modern form became popular in western countries starting in the 1960s as part of increased interest in health food and vegetarian diets. Traditional muesli was eaten with orange juice and not milk.

Serves 1–2

½ cup gluten-free oats

2 tablespoons currants

¼ cup unsweetened almond milk

¼ cup unsweetened apple juice

1 Gala or other apple, grated

1 tablespoon chia seeds

½ teaspoon apple pie spice or roasted cinnamon

½ teaspoon alcohol-free vanilla

Pour the unsweetened apple juice and unsweetened almond milk in a large glass and stir in the extract, spice, and chia seeds.

Place the oats and currants in a medium bowl. Grate the apple over the oats.

Pour the liquid mixture over the apple and oats and mix well. Place in the refrigerator covered overnight. The chia seeds will swell and become gelatinous and the next day will have absorbed all of the liquid and become almost like a pudding.

In the morning you can enjoy this dish cold or warm in the microwave. You can also add additional fruits and almond milk, if desired.

Notes: Feel free to substitute regular cinnamon for roasted. Apple pie spice is a blend of cinnamon, nutmeg, and mace. For a delicious variation, substitute a grated pear for the apple or goji berries for the currants.

Raw Chia Seed Pudding
with Cinnamon

—JOANNE WILLIAMS—

Rich in fiber, calcium, iron, and Omega-3 fatty acid (over 1 gram per serving!), you need not feel guilty about indulging in this wonderful tapioca-like pudding. Plan 30 hours ahead to allow for soaking and for the pudding to thicken.

Requires High-Speed Blender (such as a Vitamix or Blendtec)

Serves 6

½ cup raw cashews, soaked 6 hours and rinsed

3 pitted, large Medjool dates soaked 6 hours in 2¼ cups water (reserve all soak water)

1 teaspoon vanilla extract

¼ teaspoon cinnamon, plus extra for sprinkling

2 (1-gram) packets stevia powder

¼ cup chia seeds

Place the cashews, dates, date-soak water, vanilla, cinnamon, and stevia in a blender and blend until smooth and creamy.

Combine the cashew mixture with the chia seeds in a 1-quart container and stir vigorously with a fork for 1 minute.

Let the mixture sit for 15 minutes and stir again until the chia seeds are well blended and separated. Place in the refrigerator until the chia seeds absorb all of the liquid and the pudding thickens, about 24 hours.

Sprinkle with cinnamon and serve.

Sweet Potato Flatbread

—CAROLYN SCOTT-HAMILTON—

This is a wonderful gluten-free version of flatbread that might just become your favorite. It's easy to make.

Serves 4–6

Non-stick cooking spray

2 medium sweet potatoes (skinned, cooked and mashed)

1½ cups almond, quinoa or chickpea flour

2 flax eggs (2 tablespoons ground flax seeds mixed with 4 tablespoons water until gel-like)

½ cup shredded vegan mozzarella cheese

1 tablespoon nutritional yeast

1 teaspoons baking powder

1–2 teaspoons fresh minced garlic

1 teaspoon dried oregano flakes

½ teaspoon dried parsley flakes

½ teaspoon crushed red pepper flakes (optional)

1 teaspoon salt

Preheat oven to 375°F. Combine all ingredients in a large bowl, mixing well until fully incorporated.

Coat a foil lined pizza pan or baking sheet with non-stick cooking spray.

Using a spatula, spread the dough evenly into a large circle if using a pizza pan about ½-inch thick, or a rectangle if using the baking sheet.

Bake for 30 minutes until center is firm and edges are lightly browned.

Remove crust from oven, if making pizza, add toppings of choice, and bake for another 5–7 minutes. If using as crostini or breadsticks, remove from oven, brush with herbed olive oil or vegan butter, cut into slices or wedges, and bake for an additional 3 minutes.

Creamy Ginger-Hemp Dressing

—JILL NUSSINOW—

This dressing has sparkle. It was inspired by a recipe by Carrie Forrest of CarrieOnVegan.com. Use on top of grain or green salads or any time it tastes good to you.

Makes 1 cup

¼ cup shelled hemp seeds

2 tablespoons red onion

1-inch piece fresh ginger, peeled

1 teaspoon citrus zest

⅓ cup fresh citrus juice — lime, lemon or orange

½ large pitted Medjool date

¼ cup vegetable broth

1–2 teaspoons white, or other, miso

1 teaspoon tamari or *Bragg Liquid Aminos*

Combine hemp seeds, onion and ginger in the high speed blender. Whir for about 15 seconds. Add the remaining ingredients and process until smooth and creamy.

Hemp Seed Chocolate Mylk

—SHARON GREENSPAN—

Making your own non-dairy mylk takes minutes and costs pennies! You can substitute other nuts or seeds. I like to use hemp seeds since it contains all the essential amino acids and essential healthy fats (Omega-3, 6, 9). If you substitute almonds, it's best to soak them overnight (or all day) to make them more digestible and less gas producing. Some people peel the almonds to eliminate the tannins in the skin. Others do not bother. This recipe is a winner — especially with kids!

Serves 4–6

½ cup shelled hemp seeds

1 quart (4 cups) water

½ cup raw cacao powder

½ cup coconut nectar

1 heaping tablespoon vanilla powder

Blend hemp seeds and water in a high speed blender. Strain through a cheese cloth bag and return liquid to blender container.

Add remaining ingredients and blend until smooth. Store in the refrigerator for 2–3 days. If liquid separates, just shake.

Macadamia Yellow Cheese

—SHARON GREENSPAN—

The creaminess of macadamia nuts makes this a winner with any crowd! Fermenting the cheese will add probiotics — making digestion easier, improving your digestive health and strengthening your immune system. If you want to make it for immediate consumption use ¼ cup water instead of 2 cups and ¼ teaspoon of salt instead of ½ teaspoon. You can also substitute different nuts and seeds for a variety of flavors and textures.

Serves 4–6

1 cup organic raw macadamia nuts

1 cup organic raw walnuts

Ample water to cover nuts for soaking

½ teaspoon salt (sea, Celtic or Himalayan)

1 teaspoon turmeric

2 teaspoons organic sundried tomato

2 tablespoons organic lemon juice

2 cups clean water

Put the nuts in a jar and soak overnight (or all day). You will not see tails. Strain.

Put all ingredients and clean water in a blender. Blend on low or pulse a few times, and then blend on high until it becomes paste.

Put into a jar and cover with cheesecloth. There will be expansion as the cheese ferments, so be sure to leave an extra inch. You may want to sprinkle a little salt on top. Allow to sit at room temperature overnight (or all day). Liquid will sink to the bottom and the cheese will rise to the top.

Remove cheesecloth and eat! Spoon the cheese out of the jar. You may ingest or discard the liquid. Store leftovers tightly covered for 3–5 days in the refrigerator.

Decadent Chocolate Peanut Butter Truffles

—CAROLYN SCOTT-HAMILTON—

Once firm, roll into small truffle sized balls. Use a toothpick to dip truffles into glaze (recipe below), coat well and place on wax paper lined cookie sheet, making sure to remove the toothpick carefully. Cover holes with some extra chocolate and dust with extra cocoa powder. Chill for 10 minutes or so and enjoy! You can line an airtight container with wax paper and store in the refrigerator or freezer.

Makes about 20 truffles, depending upon their size

1 cup finely crushed peanuts

½ cup unsalted peanut butter

¼ cup cocoa powder

¼ cup fresh dates (if dry, soak for an hour or so and drain)

2 tablespoons agave syrup (add more if you want to sweeten more)

1 teaspoon vanilla extract

Pinch of sea salt

CHOCOLATE GLAZE COATING

1 cup cocoa butter, finely chopped

½ cups cocoa powder

¼ cup agave or date syrup

pinch of sea salt

¼ teaspoon vanilla extract

Put all ingredients, except for the ground peanuts, into food processor or blender until well incorporated and "pasty." Taste test for sweetness and add a bit more agave to reach desired taste. Mix in peanuts then place mixture in refrigerator and chill until firm.

For Chocolate Glaze Coating: Place cocoa butter in a double boiler to melt for 1–2 minutes. Remove from heat before all the pieces have melted. Add remaining ingredients to the pan and stir until smooth and well combined, then remove from double boiler.

Green Beans with Nut Cream Dressing
on Minced Tomato Salad

—LINDA LONG—

What a wonderful way to dress up green beans.

Serves 4

½ cups raw nuts, (peanuts, almonds, or cashews)

¼ teaspoon garlic, minced

½ cup hot water, slightly more if needed for consistency

¼ teaspoon red wine vinegar or to taste

1/8 teaspoon salt, and dash of pepper

Green beans, fresh, 4–6 ounces or 52 pieces, 2-inches each

¼ cup water

¼ teaspoon salt

1 cup tomatoes, fresh, very finely chopped, about 8 ounces

1½ tablespoon soft sun-dried tomatoes, very finely chopped

1 tablespoon onions, very finely chopped

2 teaspoons chives, very finely chopped (or parsley)

2 teaspoons brown rice vinegar (optional: rice vinegar)

¼ teaspoon salt, and dash of pepper

Nut Creamy Dressing: Add nuts and garlic to a blender, cover with very hot water and replace lid to soak while prepping the rest of the recipe. Later, blend on high until super creamy, at least a full minute. It should have thickness to bind to the green beans. If too thick add water. Add some salt and pepper. Test taste with a green bean.

Green Beans: Bring the small amount of water to a boil in a saucepan, add salt and washed green beans. Cover to cook and steam, lowering heat to medium. If you have a steaming basket it is fine to use that as well. After 5 minutes check for crisp tender. Do not overcook. Prepare a bowl of ice water as they cook. Drain the beans and add to the bowl to stop cooking and to cool. Drain and blot dry with a kitchen towel. Set aside.

Tomato Salad: If sun-dried tomatoes are not soft and fresh, soak in hot water in a covered bowl while you prep the rest of the tomato salad. Combine all the very finely chopped tomatoes, onions, and chives in a bowl. Drizzle with the vinegar.

Finish nut cream as above. Place the green beans in a bowl, drizzle with the finished nut cream to coat.

To Serve: Divide green beans and tomato salad into fours. Smooth a layer of the tomato salad to cover each salad plate. Place 13 green beans in a pile in the middle of the tomato salad allowing the edges to show. Eat and notice all the flavor!

Spicy Peanut Citrus Sauce

—JILL NUSSINOW—

This tasty sauce is wonderful over plain cooked vegetables and rice or over soba noodles and vegetables. This sauce will keep for a few days but I doubt that it will last that long. Feel free to double or triple the recipe.

Makes about 2/3 cup

- 3 tablespoons orange juice
- 2 tablespoons lime juice
- 1 teaspoon grated ginger
- ¼ cup smooth or chunky peanut butter, your choice
- 1 tablespoon reduced-sodium tamari or soy sauce
- 1 tablespoon rice vinegar
- 1–2 teaspoons toasted sesame oil or 1 teaspoon tahini
- 1 teaspoon chili paste with garlic
- 1 tablespoon finely chopped green onions
- 2 teaspoons maple syrup
- 2 tablespoons chopped roasted peanuts

Mix all ingredients together in a small bowl or shake well in a small jar, whisking if you need to.

Pumpkin Seed and Chocolate Chip Oatmeal Breakfast Bars

—DREENA BURTON—

These are a terrific "on-the-go" healthy breakfast, but perfect snack anytime of the day. Our whole family loves them!

Makes 12–16 bars

1½ cups rolled oats

1¼ cups oat flour

3–4 tablespoons pumpkin seeds

2–3 tablespoons non-dairy chocolate chips (mini chips are great if you have them, can also substitute raisins or cranberries)

1 teaspoon cinnamon

⅛ to ¼ teaspoon freshly grated nutmeg

¼ teaspoon sea salt

⅓ cup brown rice syrup

1–2 tablespoons pure maple syrup

¼ cup plus 2 tablespoons plain unsweetened non-dairy milk

Preheat oven to 350°F. In a large bowl, combine the rolled oats, oat flour, pumpkin seeds, chocolate chips or raisins (or both!), cinnamon, nutmeg, and salt. In a smaller bowl, combine the brown rice syrup with the maple syrup and milk. Add the wet ingredients into the dry mixture, stirring until well combined. Transfer the mixture to an 8-inch x 8-inch baking dish (brownie pan) lined with parchment paper, and press it down until evenly distributed. Using a sharp knife, cut to mark out the bars before you bake them to make it easier to fully cut and remove the bars once baked. (I usually mark out 16 bars, but you can make whatever size you like.) Bake for 20 minutes, then remove and let cool in pan. Once cool, use a sharp knife to fully cut the bars, then remove with a spatula.

Note: I first made these bars with just raisins, and they were delicious. Then, I tried a combination of pumpkin seeds and chocolate chips. Something about that duo really hit the mark for me, so I switched up the recipe with these as the "default"! You can always try out other add-ins to replace the pumpkin seeds/chips, such as sunflower seeds, hemp seeds, unsweetened coconut, and other dried fruit (chopped, if needed).

Pepita Parsnip Paté

—ROBIN ASBELL—

Roasted parsnips give the paté a sweet, earthy base, and a creaminess that makes it seem very rich. Toasted pumpkin seeds (pepitas) are nutty and delicious, and deserve a place in your spreads and dips repertoire. This makes a great sandwich, bruschetta, or cracker topping.

Makes 2½ cups, 4–6 servings

- 3 cups cubed peeled parsnips, 2 large
- 3 cloves garlic, peeled
- 1 teaspoon extra virgin olive oil, or vegetable stock
- 1 cup hulled pumpkin seeds (pepitas)
- ½ cup Italian parsley, washed and dried
- 1 teaspoon red miso
- 1 teaspoon rice vinegar
- ½ teaspoon salt
- ½ teaspoon cracked black pepper
- 1 tablespoon vegetable stock

Preheat the oven to 450°F. In a loaf pan or 8-inch x 8-inch pan, toss the parsnips, garlic, and olive oil or stock. Cover with foil and roast for 30 minutes, then uncover and pierce a parsnip with a paring knife. It should be very soft, if not, roast 10 minutes more. Uncover and cool.

In a large skillet, heat the pumpkin seeds over high heat until they are toasted and start to pop. It should take under five minutes. Dump the hot seeds into the food processor. Add the parsley and process until the seeds are ground. Add the roasted parsnips and miso and process until smooth. Add the vinegar, salt and black pepper, and process. Add vegetable stock with the machine running.

Hazelnut Sesame Bars

—KATJA HEINO—

Homemade snack bars are great for on-the-go snacking. These nutrient-rich goodies will keep you fueled up for hours. I use soaked and dehydrated raw hazelnuts for this recipe to increase the digestibility of the nuts. And if you prefer smaller treats, you can easily roll these into little snack balls. Store in the refrigerator as they become soft at room temperature.

Makes 9-12 bars (depending on how big you cut them)

1 cup dates, pitted

½ cup coconut butter, melted

2 tablespoons almond butter

3 tablespoons filtered water

¼ teaspoon celtic sea salt

1 cup hazelnuts, raw

2 tablespoons sesame seeds

In food processor, process dates, coconut butter, almond butter, salt, and water until they form a paste. Add hazelnuts and pulse until nuts are broken down into tiny bits. Add sesame seeds and pulse to combine. You may need to add a bit of water here. Mixture should be tacky but not sticky wet. Add water a tiny bit at a time.

Press mixture firmly into a 9-inch x 11-inch baking pan that is lined with parchment paper. Use the back of your spatula or your fingers to even out the top.

Place in freezer for about an hour then remove and cut into desired sized bars.

Store in fridge, separating layers with parchment paper.

No-Bean Hummus

—KAREN RANZI—

Most people cannot guess that there are no beans in this dish because it tastes so good.

Serves 4–6

2 cups peeled zucchini, chopped

½ cup hulled sesame seeds

Juice of one lemon

1 clove garlic (optional)

1 teaspoon paprika

Blend all ingredients until smooth. Serve at room temperature or chilled.

Herbed Sesame Crackers

—KAMI MCBRIDE—

These crackers are delicious as a garnish on salads and crumbled into soups. Not only are they great for dipping into hummus and veggie spreads, but because of their delicious taste, they are a great snack by themselves. You can add more cayenne if you like a spicier cracker.

Serves 4–6 or more

2 cups flax seeds	3 cloves garlic
1½ cups sesame seeds	2 tablespoons tomato paste
3 cups water	¼ cup lemon juice
1 teaspoon salt	2 tablespoons organic tamari
¼ cup apple cider vinegar	1 teaspoon cumin
3 stalks celery	1 teaspoon coriander
2 carrots	1 teaspoon paprika
1 cup parsley	¼ teaspoon cayenne
½ cup chopped onion	1 teaspoon salt

Soak the flax, sesame, water, salt and vinegar in a bowl overnight.

Put celery, carrots, onions, parsley, garlic and spices into a food processor and pulse until everything is chopped and mixed well.

Mix all ingredients along with soaked seeds into a *Vitamix* or large blender. Blend until everything is mixed well into a broth like consistency. Let broth sit for one hour then pour onto sheets and dehydrate in the dehydrator for 8 to 12 hours or until the crackers are to your liking.

Gomasio
Seaweed, Seeds and Salt Sprinkle
—JILL NUSSINOW—

This blend can be any combination that includes sea vegetables but usually has salt and sesame seeds as well. Here we will use the seaweed-dulse. To make it even more flavorful, toast the sesame seeds in a dry pan for 2–3 minutes over medium heat. Let cool before mixing with other ingredients.

Makes ¼ cup

3 tablespoons ground dried dulse, or other dried seaweed

½ teaspoon salt

1 tablespoon flax or black sesame seeds, or a combination, toast the sesame seeds only

Combine well and use on top of rice or other dishes. Because this blend has sesame or flax seeds, it has a shorter shelf life than some other blends.

"Maizing" Brassica Pizza

—MARK SUTTON—

"Maize" is a ancient term for corn and in this recipe, it unites with black beans, super-vegetable mixed greens, tomatoes, peppers, onions and a creamy millet, sunflower seeds, and chili-garlic topping sauce to make a most satisfying and nutritious pizza worthy of "CHAMPions." You can save time by making the Wheat and Black Bean Dough the day before — especially easy if using a bread machine on "dough setting" — and store in your refrigerator for a few days. Let it come to room temperature before shaping into your desired pizza shape.

Wheat and Black Bean Dough
(recipe below)

Chopped mixed tender greens — kale, collards, turnip, mustard, and/or spinach (approximately 2 cups)

Sliced tomatoes (to cover pizza as desired, leave some space between slices for corn and topping sauce)

Corn — if canned, rinsed and drained (approximately 1 cup)

Mixed finely chopped fresh or dried Italian herbs (as desired)

Thinly sliced mixed sweet peppers — optional (approximately 1 cup)

Thinly sliced raw white or red onion (as desired)

Millet, Sunflower Seed, Chili-Garlic Sauce *(recipe below)*

Pre-heat oven to 425°F or 450°F. Assemble pizza in the order indicated above. Bake pizza 15–20 minutes, depending upon your oven. Let cool a few minutes before slicing and serving.

Notes: If greens are not tender, sauté them briefly in a no-oil liquid such as white wine, water, maybe a little balsamic vinegar for acidity, or even Vermouth. Drain, if need be, after cooking. If not using fresh tomatoes, be sure to drain and "squeeze" out some of the liquid. Raw corn kernels fresh off of the cob can be used quite nicely for extra crunch. Visually, it's most effective to use orange and red sweet peppers if available. Chopped scallions or leeks could also be used in lieu of onions.

Wheat and Black Bean Dough

Puréed black beans play a starring role as a fiber and protein-rich addition to this unique whole wheat pizza dough.

This recipes makes two finely textured 12 to 14-inch pizza crusts or 1 large crust

¾ cups black beans (about ½ of a 15-ounce can)

⅓ cup water

⅔ cups warm water

1–1¼ teaspoon sugar (or sweetener of choice)

2¼ teaspoons yeast

1½ cups unbleached whole wheat bread or all-purpose flour

1 cup unbleached whole wheat flour

½ teaspoon salt (optional)

Rinse and drain beans, then purée in a blender or food processor with ⅓ cup water until smooth. Add water as necessary (in 1 tablespoon increments).

Whisk together warm water, sugar, yeast, and bean purée.

Mix together flours and salt, add slowly to yeast mixture (if not using a bread machine, stir as flour mixture is added).

Knead until the dough is elastic, let rise, covered, for at least an hour. Shape pizza dough on a lightly oiled non-stick baking sheet.

Notes: Whether making dough by hand or with a bread machine, it might be necessary to adjust the amount of flour or water in 1 tablespoon increments to get proper elasticity (think of the firmness of an "ear lobe" as the proper texture).

Vegan Cane Sugar (available at *Whole Foods Market*), molasses, barley, and malt syrups are suitable sweeteners in equivalent measure.

Millet, Sunflower Seeds, and Chili-Garlic Sauce

Cultivated for over 10,000 years, millet is a significant source of niacin, B6, and folic acid (B vitamins), as well as magnesium, calcium, iron, and zinc. In this recipe, millet combines with tasty sunflower seeds (a good source of Vitamin E as well as pantothenic acid, phosphorus, copper, manganese and selenium) to make a thick, almost custardy "cheese-like" topping sauce .

Makes about 3 cups

2 cups cooked millet (see recipe below)

1/3 cup raw, unsalted sunflower seeds

2 tablespoons nutritional yeast (optional)

1 teaspoon garlic powder

1 teaspoon salt (optional)

3 tablespoons corn starch

1/2 tablespoon (or to taste) *Sriracha* (chili-garlic) sauce

1 3/4 to 2 cups water

To prepare millet: Combine 2/3 cup millet with 1 1/3 cup water in a pot, bring to a slow boil, then turn heat down low. Let simmer, covered, for 15–20 minutes. This recipe differs from some in that it doesn't produce a very fluffy millet. Yields about 2 cups cooked millet.

To prepare sauce: Process everything in a blender or food processor until the mixture is a smooth, thick pancake-like batter. Adding the water incrementally will help facilitate assessing the sauce's thickness as it's blending. This is a longer processing due to amount of millet being used. Pour on top of pizza fillings before baking completed pizza.

Notes: Using 1 3/4 cups of water yields a very thick sauce that makes nice "clumps" on top of a pizza, whereas more water will enable it to be poured easier from processing container.

Dijon mustard will provide a tangy taste if substituted for the *Sriracha* sauce. Leftover sauce plays well with cooked pasta, steamed vegetables, and baked potatoes. You may need to thin it some with a little liquid of choice.

Using raw cashews instead of sunflower seeds is a good substitute (although higher in oil content and a more expensive). The sauce's texture profile will be a bit heavier, while still maintaining a nice taste feel.

Grain-Free Just Seeds Crackers

—KATJA HEINO—

These delicious crackers are gluten, grain, and nut free. The recipe is so versatile that you can experiment with different seed combinations to find the flavor that you like the best. Ratios are not so important in this recipe as long as the "dough" is moist enough to stick together as you roll it out. Feel free to add any other herbs that you may have growing in the garden. And for a lighter, crispier cracker, try adding an extra tablespoon of coconut oil and decreasing the water slightly. Have fun with it.

Makes 25–30 crackers (depending on how big you cut them)

1 cup sunflower seeds, raw

½ cup sesame seeds, raw

2 tablespoons pumpkin seeds, raw

2 tablespoons flax seeds, ground

2 tablespoons hemp seeds

1 tablespoon fresh rosemary or 2 tablespoons fresh cilantro, finely chopped

½ teaspoon celtic sea salt

5 tablespoons water

1 tablespoons coconut oil, melted

Place sunflower seeds into food processor and process until ground into a coarse flour. Add pumpkin seeds and pulse several times to break up seeds. Add the rest of the ingredients and pulse until well combined and starting to stick together to form a dough.

Roll out dough between 2 pieces of parchment paper to ¼-inch (or less) thick. Score the crackers into desired sizes with a pizza cutter.

Bake at 325°F for 20–25 minutes until edges begin to brown slightly.

Allow to completely cool then gently break along cut lines.

Kale Cabbage Coleslaw
with Sunflower Seed Spicy Thai Dressing

—SHIVIE COOK—

A favorite and weekly staple when we had our private clients (we changed the dressing weekly). Softly wilted kale combines with red and green cabbage for a pretty salad that packs a nutritional punch. This is a sturdy salad that can be made ahead of time (without dressing) and will keep in the fridge for 3–4 days. Chop a lot at once and eat for days!

Makes 2 cups

COLESLAW

2 bunches kale

½ head small red cabbage finely chopped

½ head small green cabbage finely chopped

1 red bell pepper diced

1 avocado

1 apple, sliced

½ cup pomegranate seeds

Lemon juice (for apple)

Arame or hijiki seaweed, soaked for 10–20 minutes and rinsed

Crunchy sea veggies mix, if available

DRESSING

⅓ cup sesame or olive oil

⅓ cup tamari

1 cup water

¾ to 1 cup sunflower seeds

Juice of 2 limes

1 tablespoon maple syrup (optional)

2–3 teaspoons ground chile or chile flakes (or to taste, it can get spicy)

Piece of fresh ginger

Tear kale from stems into small pieces and put in bowl. Gently massage with the hands for a few minutes and watch the kale wilt before your very eyes as though it had been steamed. Add red and green cabbage. Sprinkle with diced red pepper, sliced apples, pomegranate seeds, hijiki or arame and crunchy sea veggies.

Place all dressing ingredients in a high speed blender and blend until smooth, taste for spices and adjust accordingly. Add dressing to your salad 5–30 minutes before serving; it will be wilted and delicious. Great for dressing sea veggie salad or as a dip to nori and green rolls.

When storing, keep dressing separate. Keeps 3–5 days in refrigerator.

Herbed Sunflower Seed Dip or Spread
with a Fermented "Cheeze" Variation

—JILL NUSSINOW—

This is a rich but easy to make dip. Go easy on the dip and eat it with lots of vegetables or wrapped in lettuce leaves with sprouts and tomato. Or serve on top of cucumber slices or with crackers. It can be frozen if you find that you've made too much of it.

Makes 2 cups

1 cup raw sunflower seeds

1–2 tablespoons lemon juice

2–3 tablespoons chopped Italian parsley

½ cup basil leaves

1–2 tablespoons nama shoyu or tamari

1–2 cloves garlic, minced

Freshly ground black pepper, to taste

Soak the sunflower seeds in water for at least 2 hours, or overnight, or from morning until evening.

Drain sunflower seeds (reserving water in case you need it) and put into food processor or high speed blender with the remaining ingredients. Process until smooth, scraping down the sides as you need to. Let sit at least 20 minutes for the flavors to blend.

Note: To make this even more interesting and give it probiotic qualities, you can add 2 tablespoons of truly fermented pickle or sauerkraut juice to this. Transfer to a glass jar and put a paper towel on top and secure with a rubber band. Leave at room temperature for 24–48 hours. Check to see if this has fermented after 24 hours and if it is to your liking. Then eat or refrigerate.

Cherry-Chocolate Walnut Truffles

—AMBER SHEA CRAWLEY—

These bites of heaven appear deceptively simple, containing only five ingredients, but their flavor is deep and complex: a sultry mixture of sweet, bitter, fruity, nutty, and tangy, all wrapped up in one tender little package.

Makes about 24 truffles

¾ cup dry raw walnuts

1 cup pitted dates

½ cup dried cherries

¼ cup unsweetened cocoa powder or raw cacao powder

Pinch of sea salt

Combine the walnuts and dates in a food processor. Pulse together until the nuts are finely ground and the dates are well-incorporated.

Add the cherries, cocoa powder, and salt and pulse until combined, chopping the fruit as much or as little as you wish. The mixture will be very sticky.

Scoop up the mixture a tablespoon at a time and roll into a ball between your palms. Place the balls on a plate lined with waxed paper.

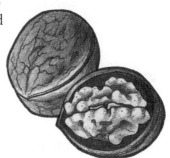

When all truffles have been formed, refrigerate for 1 hour or until ready to serve.

Raw Cinnamon Rolls

—TESS CHALLIS—

Think of these as a quick, delicious, healthy alternative to packaged energy bars. Since they're so nutrient-dense, just one little roll can be surprisingly satisfying!

Makes 4–6 servings (9 rolls)

½ cup raw walnuts

¼ cup raisins

¼ cup (packed) pitted dates (about 12 dates)

1 teaspoon cinnamon

⅛ teaspoon each: sea salt and ground nutmeg

Place all of the ingredients in a food processor. Blend until well combined and very crumbly, but don't over-blend — you want to retain some texture.

Pull out small pieces of the mixture and roll into 1-inch balls with your hands.

These will store in an airtight container, refrigerated, for several weeks or more.

Taco Nut "Meat"

—CAROLYN SCOTT-HAMILTON—

What an easy and filling way to stuff tortillas, lettuce, chard leaves or tender collard greens.

Serves 4

1 cup raw walnuts (soaked 3–4 hours and dried)

1 tablespoon ground cumin

1 tablespoon ground coriander

1 teaspoon garlic powder

1 teaspoon onion powder

1 teaspoon paprika

Pinch of cayenne

Up to ⅓ cup olive oil (optional if you want it oil free)

Salt and pepper, to taste

1 teaspoon tamari or soy sauce

Pulse walnuts in a food processor until crumbly but not pasty.

Dump walnuts into a bowl and add other ingredients, mixing until all ingredients are well incorporated, slowly adding in oil until you reach desired texture.

Use in tacos, burritos, salads and even on crackers!

To Wrap Up — The Reason for CHAMPS

NOW THAT YOU'VE LOOKED through the entire book of recipes and information, it's time to share a bit more about my eating philosophy and why eating well leads to more happiness.

I envisioned this book as a framework for providing a breadth of tasty recipes from which you can choose for your daily eating. Some recipes certainly take more time to prepare than others but I hope that you will be able to select at least ten that will make it to your menu planning rotation. (I read this on Facebook and just about fell out of my chair. In all my years of cooking, I have not ever done menu planning in that way. Still, I think that it's a good idea.) There are recipes that you might want to eat weekly, or maybe even daily. All contain the CHAMPS ingredients, and many contain foods from more than one category which can fit into a plan that provides foods that impact your health in a positive way.

When you are in good health, you generally are happier. It's hard to be in ill health and be truly happy. All the money in the world cannot buy you better health. It is completely your responsibility to choose the best-for-you foods whenever possible. I dare not say all the time because sometimes life circumstances get in the way. At home, though, there are no excuses for not eating well. It's your food sanctuary and your opportunity to provide optimal nutrition, along with great flavor which will provide the energy you need to fuel your body and brain. That is what will keep you feeling energetic and happy. It's all one big circle or cycle.

I want to see you function at your peak performance. It's why I do what I do. I already know how to eat well but there is no joy in keeping it to myself. I want to share with you, as I have with thousands of other people over my many years in the nutrition field.

There are no perfect people, no perfect recipes but I bring these to you with joy, love, peace and gratitude. I believe that you need to pay attention to what you put in your mouth. With the same level of importance, consider what comes out of your mouth. Kindness, compassion and love are important in my life. I hope that you will embrace these values too.

Absolutes don't work for me. I am not wrong and you are "right," or vice versa. Learn, explore, change, be flexible and give yourself room to be imperfect. My yoga teacher says, "We are all perfect in our imperfection." I agree.

So, back to the food, as I can wax poetic about life on my blog or elsewhere.

Here are my final thoughts about food and eating well. I promised in the title of this book that it would be a guide to both eating and cooking.

I realize that the spectrum of plant-based eating can be confusing. One person uses tamari like it's water but thinks that nuts are "bad." Another is sugar, salt and oil-free but thinks that soy is OK. Someone else declares that soy is the devil. What about seeds? They're for the birds. Don't touch avocado as it is too fattening. Moderation? It kills. What are you to believe? That is a personal decision but I hope to give you some guidance.

Avoid micromanaging your food if, and when, you can. Decide what's on your to-eat list and what's on your to-avoid list. Stick to this as often as possible. Keep "problem" foods out of the house or any of your environments: the car, the office. You know what I mean.

My best practices and advice (Embrace it or not. As they say in AA, take what you want and leave the rest):

Buy foods in the least processed form imaginable, as whole foods. Packaged, processed or fast food should not make up the bulk of what you eat. Avoid flour and white products such as sugar, rice, pasta and salt.

Buy in bulk, if you can, and buy from local farmers and producers. Even better, grow your own. Avoid *genetically modified organisms* (GMOs). Buy organic when you can (or if you choose to).

Let's all agree to eat more vegetables, especially those that are cruciferous which probably includes some that you already like, some you want to like and some you want to try. Read "Chapter One: Cruciferous Vegetables," starting on page 1 for ideas.

A recent study in *The Journal of Epidemiology and Community Health* showed a strong association between eating seven servings of vegetables and fruit a day with a 25% lower risk of dying from cancer, and a 31% lower risk of dying from heart disease or stroke during the study period. Vegetables seemed to provide a greater health benefit than fruit.

Eating vegetables and fruit n season is better for you and the environment, and they taste better. We don't have to ship food halfway around the world or across the country to get it. Yes, I live in California. Yes, we have more options here but if I had to, I could live on cabbage and root vegetables most of the winter. If we have a freeze, the price of lettuce skyrockets so I switch to cabbage or other greens. I grow sprouts (see Resources for sprout seeds).

Eating simply makes your life simpler. Make food and freeze it so that you don't have to cook every day. This book gives you so many choices for upping the cooking game.

Some people like to convert *Standard American Diet* (SAD) foods to "better and healthier" versions but how much better are they? My 76-year-old vegan friend Rick says, "It's food. How good does it need to be?" Only you know the answer.

When looking for tasty and nutritious choices upon which to build your daily eating, eat the CHAMPS way, for your health and happiness.

—Jill Nussinow

Robin Asbell: Author of *Sweet and Easy Vegan Treats Made with Whole Grains and Natural Sweeteners* (Chronicle Books, Fall 2012) *Big Vegan* (Chronicle Books) and blogging, posting free recipes and events at: www.robinasbell.com.

Beverly Lynn Bennett: Vegan chef, cookbook author, and host of the popular website: The Vegan Chef (www.veganchef.com). She lives in Eugene, Oregon. Her latest cookbook is *Chia: Using the Ancient Superfood* (Book Publishing Company 2014).

Dreena Burton: Recipe from *Plant-Powered 15*. Dreena is the author of vegan cookbooks including *Let Them Eat Vegan*. For more recipes, visit her online at: www.plantpoweredkitchen.com.

Leslie Cerier: "The Organic Gourmet," internationally recognized Farm to Table chef, educator, recipe developer, caterer, TV guest chef/presenter, health coach and author of 6 cookbooks specializing in local, seasonal, organic vegetarian, and gluten-free cooking for health, vitality, and pleasure. Find her online at: www.lesliecerier.com

Tess Challis: A vegan chef, cooking instructor, and wellness coach. She's also the author of four cookbooks. Tess has been vegan since 1991 and her greatest passion is helping others become vibrantly healthy while still enjoying the most delicious foods on the planet! Find her online at: www.radianthealth-innerwealth.com

Shivie Cook: Author of *Loving Yourself Now*. Find her online at: www.lovingyourselfnow.com

Fran Costigan: Recipes adapted from *More Great Good Dairy Free Desserts Naturally,* Book Publishing Company, 2006. Visit the author and check out her newest book, *Vegan Chocolate: Unapologetically Luscious and Decadent Dairy-Free Desserts,* Running Press, 2013, Find her online at: www.francostigan.com

Amber Shea Crawley: Author of *Practically Raw* and *Practically Raw Desserts*. Find her online at: www.chefambershea.com

Morgan Eccleston: A food blogger from *Fo' Reals Life* (www.forealslife.com) is passionate about proving that healthy plant based foods can and should taste amazing. She especially enjoys recreating healthier versions of childhood comfort foods for her friends and family.

JL Fields: A vegan cook, lifestyle coach and educator, and writes the blog: www.jlgoesvegan.com. She is the author of *Vegan Pressure Cooking* and co-authorof *Vegan for Her: The Woman's Guide to Being Healthy and Fit on a Plant-Based Diet.*

Cathy Fisher: A plant-based cooking instructor who teaches at True North Health Center and the McDougall Program in Santa Rosa, CA. To view her healthy plant-based recipes, visit her online at: www.StraightUpFood.com

Carrie Forrest: A former world champion of Hating to Eat Vegetables, Carrie has a masters degree in public health nutrition, is the author of the blog at: www.carrieonvegan.com and creator of the recipe app *Vegan Delish.* Find her online at: www.vegandelish.com

Camina Gillotti: An Ayurvedic Health Practitioner who focuses on preventative care by maintaining balance and connection to nature through food, lifestyle, and seasonal practices. She currently sees clients and teaches at the Center for Inner Health and Stillness in Santa Rosa, CA. You can email her at: Camina.Gillotti@gmail.com

Sharon Greenspan: A Board Certified Health Practitioner, speaker, and author. Author of *Wild Success® from Wildly Successful Fermenting.* Find her online at: www.wildsuccess.us and www.sugardetoxnow.com

Lydia Grossov: A passionate cook since she was 13 years old and a vegetarian, now vegan, for a over 21 years. She is a co-founder of *From A to Vegan:* www.fromatovegan.com and an event organizer of the *Bucks County Vegan Supper Club.* Find her online at www.meetup.com/Bucks-County-Vegan-Supper-Club

Nikki Haney: Author of *The Tolerant Vegan* Find her online at: www.TheTolerantVegan.com

Ellen Jaffe Jones: "The Veg Coach," Certified Personal Trainer and Running Coach, cooking instructor, accomplished endurance/sprint runner (7th in US W60-64 1500 meters, 10th in 400 Meters, 67 5K AG awards). She is the author of *Eat Vegan on $4 a Day,* and *Kitchen Divided, Paleo Vegan.* Find her online at: www.vegcoach.com.

Katja Heino: Author of the food and wellness blog: Savory Lotus. She focuses on REAL, unprocessed, nutrient-dense foods to nourish the body, mind, and soul and is passionate about helping people simplify their journey to health. To find gluten and grain-free recipes and healthy living tips visit her online at: www.savorylotus.com.

Kathy Hester: Author of *The Vegan Slow Cooker, The Great Vegan Bean Book, Vegan Slow Cooking for Two or just You* and her latest book, *OATrageous Oatmeals* is full of savory and sweet oatmeal and comes out Fall of 2014.

Chef AJ: Author of *Unprocessed* and co-producer of "Healthy Taste of LA" events. She has followed a plant-based diet for more than 35 years and is proud to say that her IQ is higher than her cholesterol. Find her online at: www.eatunprocessed.com

Ellen Kanner: Author of *Feeding the Hungry Ghost: Life, Faith and What to Eat for Dinner* and *Huffington Post's Meatless Monday* blogger. Find her online at: www.ellen-ink.com

Jaime Karpovich: Emmy-nominated host of *Save the Kales!,* a vegan television show based in the Lehigh Valley, PA airing since 2012. The show includes body-positivity, inspiration, and community activism by blending plant-based cooking with interviews from community artists, small business owners and everyday revolutionaries. She is a public speaker and freelance writer. Find her online at: www.savethekales.com

Judith Kingsbury: publisher, writer, editor, cook and photographer for *Savvy Vegetarian* since 2003. She is the mother of 3 daughters, grandmother of 7, loves meditating, reading, gardening, dancing, art, music, and travel. Judith went vegan in 2008, so now *Savvy Vegetarian* is vegan, but all are welcome. *Savvy Vegetarian* supports vegans, vegetarians, semi-veg or anyone moving toward a plant-based diet. Find her online at www.savvyvegetarian.com

Linda Long: food photographer and author of *Virgin Vegan: The Meatless Guide to Pleasing Your Palate,* and *Great Chefs Cook Vegan*. Find her online at: www.lindalong.com

Jenn Lynskey: Find her online at: www.vegandance.blogspot.com

Kami McBride: A teacher of herbal medicine since 1988. She empowers people to use herbal medicine in their daily lives for home wellness care. Kami is the author of *The Herbal Kitchen* and can be found online at: www.livingawareness.com

Mary McDougall: Author of the recipes in *The Starch Solution,* as well as many other McDougall best-selling books. Information on The McDougall Program, many free starch-based recipes, and healing your body through healthy eating can be found online at: www.drmcdougall.com.

Victoria Moran: Author of *Main Street Vegan*, praised by Michael Moore and Bill Clinton. She hosts the *Main Street Vegan* podcast and heads *Main Street Vegan Academy,* training Vegan Lifestyle Coach/Educators. Find her online at: www.mainstreetvegan.net

Christy Morgan: Author of *Blissful Bites: Plant-based Meals That Nourish Mind, Body, and Planet.* Christy's online wellness and fitness programs allow you to transform your life, reboot your health, and reach your fitness goals from anywhere in the world. Find her online at: www.theblissfulchef.com

Lani Muelrath, MA: The author of *The Plant-Based Journey: A Step-By-Step Guide for Transitioning to a Healthy Lifestyle and Achieving Your Ideal Weight* (Ben Bella, 2015) and *Fit Quickies: 5 Minute Targeted Body Shaping Workouts.* More resources online at: www.lanimuelrath.com

Joanne Mumola Williams, PhD: The author of the eBook, *Health Begins in the Kitchen,* and the creator of the blog: www.FoodsForLongLife.com. She lives in Sebastopol, CA where she and her husband grow and make Pinot Noir wines.

Heather Nicholds: A registered Holistic Nutritionist, Heather shows you how to have fun while making simple, fast, healthy and incredibly delicious meals that leave you and your family satisfied and full of energy. She creates meal plans, teaches cooking classes and does online consultations. Find her online at: www.HealthyEaingStartsHere.com

Jill Nussinow aka **The Veggie Queen™** is a Registered Dietitian, cookbook author, cooking teacher and speaker. She conceived this book and is also author of *The Veggie Queen: Vegetables Get the Royal Treatment* and *The New Fast Food: The Veggie Queen Pressure Cooks Whole Food Meals in Less than 30 Minutes.* Find her online at: www.theveggiequeen.com

Gita Patel MS, RD, CDE, CLT, LD: Author of vegetarian-gluten-free-Indian cooking, *Blending Science with Spices: Tasty Recipes and Nutrition tips for Healthy Living.* Available in print and electronic formats online at: www.feedinghealth.com

Karen Ranzi: Author of *Raw Food Fun for Families.* Find her online at: www.superhealthychildren.com

Rita Rivera: Author of *Milks Alive: 140 recipes for Plant-based Milks from a Variety of Nuts and Seeds,* Rita has a varied background in the performing arts, the healing arts, entrepreneurship. Find her online at: www.MilksAlive.com

Robin Robertson: Author of more than 20 cookbooks including, *Vegan Planet, 1,000 Vegan Recipes, One-Dish Vegan, Vegan on the Cheap,* and *Quick-Fix Vegan.* Find her online at: www.RobinRobertson.com

Elisa Rodriguez: A registered dietitian specializing in autoimmune illnesses, Elisa teaches clients how to enrich their health by taking a holistic and integrative approach. Find her online at: www.eaturveggies.com.

Miyoko Schinner: Author, speaker, television cooking host, Miyoko is the author of *Artisan Vegan Cheese* (Book Publishing Co., 2012), *The Homemade Vegan Pantry: The Art of Making Your Own Staples* (Ten Speed Press 2014).

Carolyn Scott-Hamilton: A bilingual, healthy and green living and travel expert, TV show host, vegan chef, holistic nutritionist, cookbook author, consultant, speaker and creator of the website: www.healthyvoyager.com

Mark Sutton: An accomplished speaker, avid nature photographer, gardener, and environmentalist, and self-published author of the first vegan pizza cookbook, *Heart Healthy Pizza: Over 100 Plant-Based Recipes for the Healthiest Pizza in the World.* His recipes are mostly gluten-free. He can be reached online at: www.hearthealthypizza.com

Laura Theodore: Host and creator of the PBS award-winning, vegan cooking series, *Jazzy Vegetarian.* She is author of Jazzy Vegetarian Classics: *Vegan Twists on American Family Favorites* and *Jazzy Vegetarian: Lively Vegan Cuisine That's Easy and Delicious.* For more information visit her online at: www.JazzyVegetarian.com

Amie Valpone, HHC, AADP: A Manhattan-based personal chef and culinary nutritionist, Amie is Editor-in-Chief of the website www.TheHealthyApple.com which specializes in gluten-free recipes. Amie healed herself from years of chronic pain; she shares her story of how "Clean Eating" saved her life and inspires you to clean up your food.

Jason Wyrick: Executive chef of *The Vegan Taste* and founder of the world's first vegan food magazine, *The Vegan Culinary Experience.* He is the author of *Vegan Tacos,* and the co-author of a *New York Times* best-selling book, *21-Day Weight Loss Kickstart* with Neal Barnard, MD. Find him online at: www.thevegantaste.com

Erin Wysocarski: Author and blogger at: www.olivesfordinner.com

Agar Agar: A seaweed gelatin that is used for its thickening properties. It must be cooked to be effective. It comes in powder, flakes or bars. Use what is called for in your recipe. It has a very long shelf life.

Arrowroot: From the arrowroot plant, this starch is often used as a thickener instead of the more highly processed cornstarch. Mix arrowroot powder with cool liquid, stirring well and add to food in a pan that is removed from the heat to avoid clumping. Purchase in bulk for the best price.

Asefetida aka Hing: Pronounced: *as-sah-FEH-teh-dah,* This plant grows mainly in Iran and India. The root is harvested and ground into a powder. It has a strong onion-garlic flavor and is used in small quantities to Indian dishes and spice mixes. It is stinky so be sure to store it in a well-sealed container in a dark place.

Bragg Liquid Aminos: Use in the same way as tamari or soy sauce. It is salty, contains amino acids, is not fermented and is derived from soybeans. It is also gluten-free.

Chipotle Chile: This is a smoked pepper, most often a jalapeno although *Tierra Vegetables* (see "Ingredient Sources" on pages 244-245) smokes many different types of peppers. You can buy the dried peppers whole and then process them in a spice grinder or buy the chipotle powder which is already ground. You can substitute canned chipotle peppers in adobo sauce if you must although they often contain vinegar or other seasonings. If you use canned chipotles, drain them from the sauce.

Lemongrass: The stalk of a lemongrass plant. Find it in Asian groceries, natural food stores and some supermarkets. When using it, remove some of the outer stalk. Then bruise the stalk by carefully hitting it with the blunt part of your knife. Cut into 1-inch or larger pieces. Be sure to fish these out after cooking, as they are woody and tough. You can use a bit of grated lemon zest or dried lemongrass to replicate the flavor.

Miso: A fermented soybean paste, which is very salty. There are many types and brands of miso, and the flavor of each differs. Use it sparingly or it can overpower your food. *Westbrae* or *Eden* brands are commonly available, although *South River Miso* brand is extremely delicious and more delicate. Add miso only at the end of cooking soup or stews as it has probiotic activity (beneficial bacteria) that is inactivated when cooked over heat.

Nutritional yeast: A yellow powder or flake used as a dietary supplement (B vitamins) and seasoning. It has a nutty, cheesy taste and is easily added to soups, stews, gravies, salad dressings or sauces. It is not the same as brewer's or baking yeast and the three cannot be used interchangeably. Purchase it in bulk at natural food stores and store in the refrigerator.

Silken Tofu: Made by *Mori Nu.* Silken tofu currently comes in a 12.3-ounce aseptic box that is shelf-stable and good for up to a year from the date it's made. Once opened the tofu must be refrigerated. To keep it fresh in the refrigerator for up to one week, change the water the tofu is kept in daily. I use silken tofu only for blending in soups, sauces, or dressings, not for braises, stir-fries or for baking, as it adds creaminess to recipes when blended and tends to crumble when used for other purposes. See tofu entry for what I like for other cooking.

Soy Sauce: Traditionally made soy sauce is often called shoyu. It is generally not gluten-free. Read the labels on soy sauce to see what they contain. Get the ones without salt and caramel coloring. Soy sauce can be used interchangeably with tamari or *Bragg Liquid Aminos.*

Spanish Smoked Paprika (Pimentón): It is often available in gourmet, or cooking, stores. This adds a smoky flavor to foods. It comes in mild and hot. Choose the one that works best for you. It is also available from *Whole Spice* and *Mountain Rose Herbs* (see "Ingredient Sources" on pages 244-245).

Sucanat: Natural sugar cane juice. It is unrefined and substitutes one to one for sugar, although the color is darker. It is sweet so use sparingly, as you would sugar.

Tahini: Raw or roasted sesame seed paste. I prefer raw but buy what you can find in jars or cans at the natural food store, supermarket or Middle Eastern grocery.

Tamari: A dark, wheat-free sauce made from fermented soybeans. The flavor is much better than standard soy sauce, which is mostly salt, water and coloring. Japanese shoyu is a good substitute although it contains wheat. I often use *San-J Reduced Sodium Tamari* since it is widely available at most natural food stores and some supermarkets.

Tempeh: A fermented soybean cake with origins in Indonesia where they have used it for several hundred years. It has more fiber and is less processed than tofu, with a nutty taste and firm texture. You can buy it in natural food stores and some supermarkets. You will often find it in the freezer case or the refrigerated section of the store. Once opened it must be refrigerated and can be refrozen to use later. If your tempeh gets colors or has an off-smell, toss it. Tempeh can be substituted in many recipes that call for firm tofu.

Tofu: If tofu is new to you, this information will be helpful. If you are already familiar with using tofu, read this only for a refresher. For most cooking, and especially pressure cooking, I prefer to use a firm or extra firm tofu, in a vacuum-packed refrigerated container rather than those found in water. You might need to drain or squeeze some water out of the tofu, depending upon its consistency. If the tofu is somewhat firm, you can do this by actually squeezing the tofu gently between your hands. Alternatively, you can lay the tofu on a cutting board set on an angle next to the sink and put another board on top to create pressure and let the liquid drain out for at least 15 minutes. I prefer very firm tofu that does not need that treatment but sometimes all you can get is a less firm tofu. In that case, remove as much liquid as possible. In the pressure cooker, tofu gets firmer as it cooks. It is a wonderful source of soy protein.

Vegetable Cooking Spray: This usually refers to a spray oil product such as *Pam®*. I prefer putting the oil of my choice, usually canola, olive or a combination of the two, in a spray bottle such as a *Misto®* sprayer. Most commercial sprays contain lecithin, which burns at a lower temperature than oil and can make your cookware permanently sticky. Using spray oil helps you cut down on the amount of fat that you use in cooking.

Zest: The outer, colored part of the peel on citrus fruit. Use any but grapefruit since it is too bitter. It has anti-cancer properties and adds incredible flavor with no fat. Avoid the white pith under the peel, as it is bitter. Use only organic fruit when zesting. The best way to do this is with a tool called a zester or a *Microplane™* fine grater.

If you don't live near a major city, you might find it easier to get some ingredients by mail order or online. This short list will give you a good start.

Goldmine Natural Foods

Carries a wide selection of beans, grains, miso and other macrobiotic and natural food items.

www.goldminenaturalfoods.com (800) 475-3663

Gourmet Mushrooms/Mycopia

Located in Northern California, they offer a variety of fresh and dried mushrooms, growing kits and medicinal mushroom products, sold widely.

www.mycopia.com (707) 823-1743 or (800) 789-9121

Mountain Rose Herbs

Offers a many different bulk organic herbs and spices.

www.mountainroseherbs.com (800) 879-3337

Purcell Mountain Farms

Also offers a range of rice, as well as a large assortment of lentils and conventional and organic beans, as well as spices, dried mushrooms and mushroom powders.

www.purcellmountainfarms.com (208) 267-0627

Rancho Gordo

Offers more than 20 varieties of heirloom beans, dried posole (hominy), wild rice, Mexican oregano, chiles and chile powders, and more.

www.ranchogordo.com (707) 259-1935

South River Miso

Made in Massachusetts has my favorite American-made miso. You might be able to find it at your local natural food store or you can order it in the non-summer months directly from them. They also sell "varietal" tamari that is incredible.

www.southrivermiso.com (413) 369-4057

Sprout House

Sells top quality sprout seeds and sprouting equipment. They offer the *Veggie Queen Mix, Veggie Queen Sprout Salad Mix* and *Cloverly Lentily Mix* which are my blends. Read through their site to see how to sprout seeds or search my website for sprouts to see how to grow them.

www.sprouthouse.com (800) 777-6887

Tierra Vegetables

Located in California, this farm grows a variety of heirloom beans each year, and also smokes chilies, turns them into chipotle, and chili powder, and makes hot sauce. They will do mail order if you call them.

www.tierravegetables.com (707) 837-8366

Whole Spice

Offers freshly ground spices in varying quantities with wonderful spice blends. A small selection of organic herbs and spices.

www.wholespice.com (707) 778-1750

Wineforest Wild Foods, Connie Green

Sells many varieties of wild mushrooms, spice rubs and wild American walnuts and pecans.

www.wineforest.com (707) 944-2334

NOTE: *Recipes from individual authors are listed by name and can be found in the pages immediately following the general index.*

A

Adzuki beans *(see Beans)*

Agar Agar *(see Sea Vegetables)*

Agave syrup
Decadent Chocolate Peanut Butter Truffles, 215
Grilled Mushroom and Spring Onion Salad with Miso Tahini Dressing, 135
Rainbow Sprout Salad, 178
Raw Almond Matcha Cakes, 199
Super Spring Salad with Zesty Orange Dressing, 77
The Veggie Queen's Raw Kale Salad, 41

Allium Broth, 95

Alliums *(see ingredients below)*

Chives
Chipotle Cauliflower Mashers, 27
Crunchy Kohlrabi Quinoa Salad, 42
Green Beans with Nut Cream Dressing on Minced Tomato Salad, 216
Tuscan Soup with a Twist, 192

Garlic
8-Minute Split Pea Soup, 187
Allium Broth, 95
Arugula and Herb Pesto, 3
Asian-Adzuki Bean Crockpot Chili, 149
Baby Leeks a la Nicoise, 104
Black Bean and Sweet Potato Hash, 152
Black Bean Collard Wraps, 153
Bok Choy, Green Garlic and Greens with Sweet Ginger Sauce, 8
Braised Green Cabbage, 20
Braised Turnip Greens with Tomatoes and Thyme, 52
Brazilian Black Bean Stew (Feijoada), 155
Broccoli with Turmeric, Ginger and Garlic, 84
Chickpea Curry, 160
Cilantro Avocado Dressing, 70
Creamy Caesar Salad Dressing, 96
Creamy Southern Soup Beans, 183
Curried Lentils and Spinach, 169
"Did You Say Green Onions?", 98

Falafel Patties, 163
Fresh Shelling Beans and Summer Vegetables, 158
Garlic, Greens, and Tofu with a Twist, 97
Garlic Herb Aioli, 99
Garlic Sesame Broccoli Salad, 99
Garlicky Lemon Spinach Salad with Sunflower Seeds, Olives and Sprouted Beans, 100
Ginger Lime Carrot Soup, 74
Hail to the Kale Salad, 38
Herbed Sesame Crackers, 221
Hummus, 165
Immune Broth, 136
Immune Power Soup, 137
Kale Apply Curry, 86
Kid's Kale, 39
Leek and Potato Soup, 106
Lemon-Pepper Arugula Pizza with White Bean Basil Sauce, 4
Lemony Lentil and Potato Chowder, 168
Lentil, Mushroom and Walnut Paté, 123
Minted Pea Soup, 179
Mushroom Oat Burgers, 145
Mushroom Un–Meatballs, 138
Mustard Greens and Gumbo, 44
Parsley Pistachio Lime Pesto, 81
Pasta with Zesty Lemon White Bean Sauce, 191
Pepita Parsnip Paté, 219
Roasted Beet Hummus with Thyme, 82
Roasted Cauliflower and Chickpea Curry, 29
Roasted Cauliflower with Arugula Pesto, 31
Rosemary Mushrooms and Kale, 127
Scalloped Turnips Casserole, 54
Simple Shiitake and Broccoli (Mock) Stir-Fry, 139
Shiitake Mushroom Asparagus Spinach Soup, 140
Smoked Trumpet Mushroom Potato Soup, 143
Smoky Collard Greens, 35
Smoky Sweet Black-Eyed Peas, 159
Spicy Black Bean Dip, 156
Split Pea and Yam Soup, 189
Sweet Potato Flatbread, 212
Taco Nut "Meat", 230
Tatsoi with Bok Choy and Mushrooms, 51
Tofu and Snow Pea Stir Fry Salad, 101
Tomatillo Black Bean Salsa, 70

White Bean Garlic Soup, 102
Wild Mushroom and Farro Stew, 131
Zesty Broccoli Rabe with Chickpeas and
   Pasta, 16
Watercress-Sage Pesto, 56

Green Onion
   Asian Bean Dip, 190
   Baked Broccoli Burgers, 10
   Black Bean and Sweet Potato Hash, 152
   Black Bean Collard Wraps, 153
   Cabbage Lime Salad with Dijon-Lime
      Dressing, 22
   Carrots Stir-fried with Mung Sprouts and
      Vegetables, 68
   Chickpea and Strawberry Summer Salad, 161
   Creamy Southern Soup Beans, 183
   "Did You Say Green Onions?", 98
   Immune Power Soup, 137
   Lemon Scented Spinach Spread, 103
   Mustard Greens, Snow Peas, Green Garlic and
      Kumquats Spring Slaw, 46
   Rice and Veggie Sushi Salad, 186
   Roasted Beet Hummus with Thyme, 82
   Rutabaga "Noodles" with Lemon Balsamic
      Tahini Sauce, 50
   Scalloped Turnips Casserole, 54
   Simple Shiitake and Broccoli (Mock)
      Stir-Fry, 139
   Tatsoi with Bok Choy and Mushrooms, 51
   Thai Bangkok Noodles, 115
   Tuscan Soup with a Twist, 192
   Umami Sun-Dried Tomato and Almond
      Burgers, 202

Leek
   Allium Broth, 95
   Baby Leeks a la Nicoise, 104
   Leek and Butternut Squash Soup, 105
   Leek and Potato Soup, 106
   Lentil-Leek Soup, 172
   Lentil, Mushroom and Walnut Paté, 123

Onion
   Allium Broth, 95
   Baked Stuffed Onions, 107
   Black Bean and Greens Quesadillas with
      Smoky Chipotle Cream, 151
   Black Bean and Sweet Potato Hash, 152
   Brazilian Black Bean Stew (Feijoada), 155

Broccoli with Turmeric, Ginger and Garlic, 84
Chickpea and Strawberry Summer Salad, 161
Chickpea Tomato Soup, 162
Curried Lentils and Spinach, 169
Curried White and Sweet Potato Pancakes with
   Fresh Fruit Chutney, 108
Easy Salsa Supper, 157
Falafel Patties, 163
Fat-Free "Forks Over Knives"-Style Onion
   Mushroom Gravy, 110
French Green Lentil Salad with Asparagus and
   Pine Nuts, 173
Fresh Shelling Beans and Summer Vegetables,
   158
Garden Bruschetta, 65
Garlic, Greens, and Tofu with a Twist, 97
Go-To Winter Medley, 112
Greek Garbanzo Bean Salad, 164
Green Beans with Nut Cream Dressing on
   Minced Tomato Salad, 216
Herbed Sesame Crackers, 221
Kidney Bean Salad with Chili-Lime Dressing, 166
Lemony Lentil and Potato Chowder, 168
Minted Pea Soup, 179
M'jeddrah, 174
Mustard Greens and Gumbo, 44
Potato and Watercress Soup with Sorrel
   Cream, 55
Red Lentil Soup with Sweet Potatoes and
   Spinach, 176
Roasted Cauliflower and Chickpea Curry, 29
Roasted Stuffed Onions with Carrot-Potato
   Purée, 113
Romaine Burritos, 201
Shiitake Mushroom Asparagus Spinach Soup,
   140
Smoky Collard Greens, 35
Smoky Sweet Black-Eyed Peas, 159
Split Pea and Yam Soup, 189
Tempeh and Wild Mushroom Stew, 141
Tomatillo Black Bean Salsa, 70
Tuscan Soup with a Twist, 192
Wild Mushroom and Farro Stew, 131

Shallot
   Coconut-Chickpea Crepes with Smoky Herbed
      Mushrooms, 122
   Thai Bangkok Noodles, 115
   Wild Mushroom Ravioli, 142

Almonds *(see Nuts)*

Almond butter
Dr. Shiroko Sokitch's Favorite Breakfast, 208
Hail to the Kale Salad, 38
Hazelnut Sesame Bars, 220
Sweet Watercress Smoothie, 57

Appetizers
Garden Bruschetta, 65
Mango, Daikon, and Avocado Spring Rolls, 49
Perfect Pesto Stuffed Mushrooms (raw), 66
Root Veggies Paté, 49
Stuffed Herb Pesto Holiday Appetizers, 67

Apple
Fresh Fruit Chutney with Mustard Seeds and
Cilantro, 109
Kale-Apple Slaw with Goji Berry Dressing, 37
Kale Apple Almond Milk, 199
Kale Apply Curry, 86
Kale Cabbage Coleslaw with Sunflower Seed
Spicy Thai Dressing, 227
Minted Pea Soup, 179
Overnight Muesli, 210
Quick Lentil and Eggplant Curry, 85
The Veggie Queen's Raw Kale Salad, 41

Apple juice
Blueberry Gel, 71
Kale Apple Almond Milk, 199
Overnight Muesli, 210

Arrowroot
Blueberry Gel, 71
Ginger-Pineapple Pudding, 76
Oyster Mushroom, Asparagus and Tofu Stir
Fry, 134
Tempeh and Wild Mushroom Stew, 141

Artichoke hearts
Garden Bruschetta, 65
Herby Italian Dressing, 80

Arugula
Arugula and Herb Pesto, 3
Roasted Turmeric Brussels Sprouts with Hemp
Seeds on Arugula, 19
Lemon-Pepper Arugula Pizza with White Bean
Basil Sauce, 4
Roasted Cauliflower with Arugula Pesto, 31
Shangri-La Soup, 5
Summer Arugula Salad with Lemon Tahini
Dressing, 6

Asparagus
Crunchy Kohlrabi Quinoa Salad, 42
French Green Lentil Salad with Asparagus and
Pine Nuts, 173
Oyster Mushroom, Asparagus and Tofu Stir
Fry, 134
Shiitake Mushroom Asparagus Spinach Soup,
140

Astragalus
Immune Broth, 136

Avocado
Cabbage Lime Salad with Dijon-Lime
Dressing, 22
Cilantro Avocado Dressing, 70
Easy Salsa Supper, 157
Kale Cabbage Coleslaw with Sunflower Seed
Spicy Thai Dressing, 227
Kidney Bean Salad with Chili-Lime Dressing, 166
Mango, Daikon, and Avocado Spring Rolls, 49
Rice and Veggie Sushi Salad, 186
Spicy Thai Dressing, 227
Shangri-La Soup, 5
The Veggie Queen's Raw Kale Salad, 41
Trumpet Mushroom and Avocado Ceviche, 144

B

Balsamic vinegar
Balsamic Glazed Herb Roasted Roots with
Kohlrabi, Rutabaga, Turnip, Chickpea
Tomato Soup, 162
Fennel, Carrots and Potatoes, 43
Jill's Mustard Blend, 78
Lentil, Mushroom and Walnut Paté, 123
Mediterranean Greens, 34
Roasted Maitake, 133
Roasted Turmeric Brussels Sprouts with Hemp
Seeds on Arugula, 19
Rutabaga "Noodles" with Lemon Balsamic
Tahini Sauce, 50
Umami Sun-Dried Tomato and Almond
Burgers, 202

Banana
Banana Nut Chia Pudding, 209
Black Bean Peanut Butter Brownies, 154
Sweet Watercress Smoothie, 57
The Veggie Queen's Husband's Daily Green
Smoothie, 40

Barley
  Barley, White Beans, and Horseradish Sauce, 25
Bars
  Hazelnut Sesame Bars, 220
  Pumpkin Seed and Chocolate Chip Oatmeal
    Breakfast Bars, 218
Basil *(see Herbs)*
Bay leaf *(see Herbs)*
Beans *(Pulses — see ingredients below)*
  Adzuki *(Azuki or Aduki)*
    Asian-Adzuki Bean Crockpot Chili, 149
    Protein Powerhouse Trifecta, 150
  Black
    Black Bean and Greens Quesadillas with
      Smoky Chipotle Cream, 151
    Black Bean and Sweet Potato Hash, 152
    Black Bean Collard Wraps, 153
    Black Bean Peanut Butter Brownies, 154
    Brazilian Black Bean Stew (Feijoada), 155
    Kale and Spring Pea Mash-up, 182
    Spicy Black Bean Dip, 156
    Tomatillo Black Bean Salsa, 70
  Cannellini
    Asian Bean Dip, 190
    Horseradish and Cannellini Bean Dip, 36
    Lemon-Pepper Arugula Pizza with White Bean
      Basil Sauce, 4
    Pasta with Zesty Lemon White Bean Sauce, 191
    Tuscan Soup with a Twist, 192
  Chickpeas
    Cabbage Lime Salad with Dijon-Lime
      Dressing, 22
    Chickpea Curry, 160
    Chickpea and Strawberry Summer Salad, 161
    Chickpea Tomato Soup, 162
    Falafel Patties, 163
    Greek Garbanzo Bean Salad, 164
    Hummus, 165
    Kale Apply Curry, 86
    Nourishing Stew, 175
    Roasted Beet Hummus with Thyme, 82
    Roasted Cauliflower and Chickpea Curry, 29
    Summer Arugula Salad with Lemon Tahini
      Dressing, 6
    Tuscan Soup with a Twist, 192
    Yam Boats with Chickpeas, Bok Choy and
      Cashew Dill Sauce, 9

  Zesty Broccoli Rabe with Chickpeas and
    Pasta, 16
  Fresh shelling *(also see Peas, Black-eyed)*
    Fresh Shelling Beans and Summer Vegetables,
      158
  Garbanzo *(see Chickpeas)*
  Great Northern *(see White)*
  Kidney
    Kidney Bean Salad with Chili-Lime Dressing, 166
    Vegan Red Beans and Rice, 167
  Lima
    Gutsy Greek Gigantes Beans with Greens,
      Oregano and Mint, 79
  Mung
    Rainbow Sprout Salad, 178
  Navy
    Pasta with Zesty Lemon White Bean Sauce, 191
  Pinto
    Creamy Southern Soup Beans, 183
    Pinto Bean Quinoa Burgers, 184
  Soybeans, green (Edamame)
    Miso Vegetable Soup, 185
    Rice and Veggie Sushi Salad, 186
  Steuben (Yellow-eye)
    Slow Cooker Yellow-Eyed Bean Soup with
      Sweet Potatoes and Greens, 193
  White
    Asian Bean Dip, 190
    Pasta with Zesty Lemon White Bean Sauce, 191
    Tuscan Soup with a Twist, 192
  White giant
    Gutsy Greek Gigantes Beans with Greens,
      Oregano and Mint, 79
Beets
  Roasted Beet Hummus with Thyme, 82
Berries, all
  Blueberry Gel, 71
  Chickpea and Strawberry Summer Salad, 161
  High-Fiber Blueberry, Pear, and Spinach
    Smoothie with Brazil Nuts, 203
  Summer Arugula Salad with Lemon Tahini
    Dressing, 6
  Sweet Watercress Smoothie, 57
  The Veggie Queen's Husband's Daily Green
    Smoothie, 40

Black-eyed Peas *(see Peas, Black-eyed)*

Black Truffles
    Truffled Celeriac Soup, 121

Bok Choy
    Bok Choy Ginger Dizzle, 7
    Sesame Bok Choy Shiitake Stir Fry, 7
    Bok Choy, Green Garlic and Greens with
       Sweet Ginger Sauce, 8
    Tatsoi with Bok Choy and Mushrooms, 51
    Yam Boats with Chickpeas, Bok Choy and
       Cashew Dill Sauce, 9

Blueberry *(see Berries, all)*

Bragg Liquid Aminos
    Asian-Adzuki Bean Crockpot Chili, 149
    Spiced Nuts, 91
    Spicy Black Bean Dip, 156
    Thai Bangkok Noodles, 115
    Wild Mushroom Ravioli, 142

Bread
    Quick-Stuffed Crimini Mushrooms, 125
    Sweet Potato Flatbread, 212

Bread Crumbs
    Baked Broccoli Burgers, 10
    Scalloped Turnips Casserole, 54

Broccoli
    Baked Broccoli Burgers, 10
    Broccoli with Turmeric, Ginger and Garlic, 84
    Creamy Dreamy Broccoli Soup, 11
    Fennel with Broccoli, Zucchini and Peppers, 12
    Miso Vegetable Soup, 185
    Mushroom Oat Burgers, 145
    Simple Shiitake and Broccoli (Mock) Stir-Fry,
       139
    Stir-Fry Toppings, 14
    Thai-Inspired Broccoli Slaw, 15

Broccoli Rabe (rapini)
    Zesty Broccoli Rabe with Chickpeas and
       Pasta, 16

Broccoli, Romanesco
    Romanesco Broccoli Sauce, 13

Brown rice *(see Rice, brown)*

Brown rice syrup
    Pumpkin Seed and Chocolate Chip Oatmeal
       Breakfast Bars, 218

Brussels Sprouts
    Cream of Brussels Sprouts Soup with Vegan
       Cream Sauce, 17
    "Brussels Sprouts — The Vegetable We Love to
       Say We Hate", 18
    Roasted Turmeric Brussels Sprouts with Hemp
       Seeds on Arugula, 19

Burgers
    Baked Broccoli Burgers, 10
    Mushroom Oat Burgers, 145
    Pinto Bean Quinoa Burgers, 184
    Umami Sun-Dried Tomato and Almond
       Burgers, 202

C

Cabbage
    Asian-Adzuki Bean Crockpot Chili, 149
    Braised Cabbage with Cumin, 73
    Braised Green Cabbage, 20
    Cabbage and Red Apple Slaw, 21
    Cabbage Lime Salad with Dijon-Lime
       Dressing, 22
    Kale Cabbage Coleslaw with Sunflower Seed
       Spicy Thai Dressing, 227
    Leek and Butternut Squash Soup, 105
    Rainbow Sprout Salad, 178
    Really Reubenesque Revisited Pizza, 23
    Simple Sauerkraut, 26

Cabbage, Napa
    Miso Vegetable Soup, 185
    Mustard Greens, Snow Peas, Green Garlic and
       Kumquats Spring Slaw, 46

Cacao/Cocoa/Carob
    Black Bean Peanut Butter Brownies, 154
    Cherry-Chocolate Walnut Truffles, 229
    Cocoa Spice Powder, 89
    Cocoa-Spice Roasted Squash, 69
    Decadent Chocolate Peanut Butter Truffles, 215
    Hemp Seed Chocolate Mylk, 213
    Pumpernickel or Rye Dough, 24
    Sweet Watercress Smoothie, 57

Capers
    Garlic Herb Aioli, 99
    Romanesco Broccoli Sauce, 13

Carrots
    8-Minute Split Pea Soup, 187
    Asian-Adzuki Bean Crockpot Chili, 149

Balsamic Glazed Herb Roasted Roots with Kohlrabi, Rutabaga, Turnip, Fennel, Carrots and Potatoes, 43
Cabbage Lime Salad with Dijon-Lime Dressing, 22
Chickpea Curry, 160
Chickpea Tomato Soup, 162
Herbed Sesame Crackers, 221
Leek and Butternut Squash Soup, 105
Lentil Coconut Spinach Soup, 170
Lentil-Leek Soup, 172
Kale-Apple Slaw with Goji Berry Dressing, 37
Miso Vegetable Soup, 185
Moroccan Vegetable Tagine, 53
Mushroom Oat Burgers, 145
Rainbow Sprout Salad, 178
Red Lentil Soup with Sweet Potatoes and Spinach, 176
Rice and Veggie Sushi Salad, 186
Roasted Stuffed Onions with Carrot-Potato Purée, 113
Root Veggies Paté, 49
Shangri-La Soup, 5
Veggie Mushroom Burgers, 129
Cauliflower
    Chipotle Cauliflower Mashers, 27
    Nourishing Stew, 175
    Raw Cauliflower Tabbouleh, 28
    Roasted Cauliflower and Chickpea Curry, 29
    Roasted Cauliflower with Arugula Pesto, 31
Cayenne (see Spices)
Celery
    8-Minute Split Pea Soup, 187
    Cabbage Lime Salad with Dijon-Lime Dressing, 22
    Chickpea Tomato Soup, 162
    Herbed Sesame Crackers, 221
    Kale-Apple Slaw with Goji Berry Dressing, 37
    Kale Apply Curry, 86
    Lentil Coconut Spinach Soup, 170
    Moroccan Vegetable Tagine, 53
    Root Veggies Paté, 49
    Spicy Red Lentil Vegetable Soup, 177
    Split Pea and Yam Soup, 189
    Vegan Red Beans and Rice, 167
Celery root
    Truffled Celeriac Soup, 121

Celery seed (see Spices)
Cheese, nondairy
    Herbed Sunflower Seed Dip or Spread with a Fermented "Cheeze" Variation, 228
    Macadamia Yellow Cheese, 214
    Mushroom Oat Burgers, 145
    Red Almond Cheese, 200
    Sweet Potato Flatbread, 212
Cherries, dried
    Cherry-Chocolate Walnut Truffles, 229
Chia seeds (see Seeds, Chia)
Chickpea flour
    Coconut-Chickpea Crepes with Smoky Herbed Mushrooms, 122
    Falafel Patties, 163
Chile powder, including chipotle (see Spices)
Chili
    Asian-Adzuki Bean Crockpot Chili, 149
Chocolate
    Pumpkin Seed and Chocolate Chip Oatmeal Breakfast Bars, 218
Chutney
    Fresh Fruit Chutney, 108
Cilantro (see Herbs)
Cinnamon (see Spices)
Cloves (see Spices)
Cocoa (see Cacao/Cocoa)
Cocoa butter
    Decadent Chocolate Peanut Butter Truffles, 215
Coconut
    Carrots Stir-Fried with Mung Sprouts and Vegetables, 68
    Crazy for Coconut, 208
    Hazelnut Sesame Bars, 220
Coconut milk
    Coconut-Chickpea Crepes with Smoky Herbed Mushrooms, 122
    Dr. Shiroko Sokitch's Favorite Breakfast, 208
    Lentil Coconut Spinach Soup, 170
    Nourishing Stew, 175
    Thai Bangkok Noodles, 115
    Thai-Inspired Broccoli Slaw, 15
    Thai Rice, Snow Pea and Mushroom Salad, 180
Coconut nectar
    Hemp Seed Chocolate Mylk, 213

Coconut palm sugar
    Creamy Cashew Almond Custard, 204
Coconut water or juice
    Hail to the Kale Salad, 38
Collard Greens
    Black Bean Collard Wraps, 153
    Collard Green and Quinoa Taco or Burrito
        Filling, 32
    Collard Greens Wrapped Rolls with Spiced
        Quinoa Filling, 33
    Mediterranean Greens, 34
    Smoky Collard Greens, 35
Corn
    Fresh Shelling Beans and Summer Vegetables,
        158
    Kidney Bean Salad with Chili-Lime Dressing, 166
Couscous
    Baked Broccoli Burgers, 10
Crackers
    Grain-Free Just Seeds Crackers, 226
    Herbed Sesame Crackers, 221
Cranberries, dried *(see Berries, all)*
Crimini Mushrooms *(see Mushrooms)*
Cucumber
    Bok Choy Ginger Dizzle, 7
    Cabbage Lime Salad with Dijon-Lime
        Dressing, 22
    Gingered Cucumber Salad, 75
    Raw Cauliflower Tabbouleh, 28
Cumin *(see Spices)*
Currants
    Overnight Muesli, 210
Curried dishes
    Chickpea Curry, 160
    Curried Lentils and Spinach, 169
    Quick Lentil and Eggplant Curry, 85
    Kale Apply Curry, 86
    Lentil Coconut Spinach Soup, 170
    Roasted Cauliflower and Chickpea Curry, 29
    Thai Bangkok Noodles, 115

D

Daikon *(see Radish)*
Dates
    Banana Nut Chia Pudding, 209
    Black Bean Peanut Butter Brownies, 154
    Cashew Almond Date Milk, 205
    Cherry-Chocolate Walnut Truffles, 229
    Cilantro Avocado Dressing, 70
    Decadent Chocolate Peanut Butter Truffles, 215
    Hail to the Kale Salad, 38
    Hazelnut Sesame Bars, 220
    Raw Chia Seed Pudding with Cinnamon, 211
    Raw Cinnamon Rolls, 230
    Smoky Sweet Black-Eyed Peas, 159
Dessert
    Black Bean Peanut Butter Brownies, 154
    Blueberry Gel, 71
    Cherry-Chocolate Walnut Truffles, 229
    Creamy Cashew Almond Custard, 204
    Decadent Chocolate Peanut Butter Truffles, 215
    Raw Almond Matcha Cakes, 199
    Raw Chia Seed Pudding with Cinnamon, 211
    Raw Cinnamon Rolls, 230
Dips
    Asian Bean Dip, 190
    Horseradish and Cannellini Bean Dip, 36
    Spicy Black Bean Dip, 156
    Wonder Spread, 207
"Dry Sautéing", 128

E

Eggplant
    Brazilian Black Bean Stew (Feijoada), 155
    Garden Bruschetta, 65
    Quick Lentil and Eggplant Curry, 85

F

Farro
    Wild Mushroom and Farro Stew, 131
Fennel
    Balsamic Glazed Herb Roasted Roots with
        Kohlrabi, Rutabaga, Turnip, Fennel, Carrots
        and Potatoes, 43
    Fennel with Broccoli, Zucchini and Peppers, 12
Fennel seeds *(see Spices)*
Flax seeds *(see Seeds, Flax)*
Flour
    Black Bean Peanut Butter Brownies, 154
    Rich Mushroom Gravy, 126
    Sweet Potato Flatbread, 212
French Green Lentils *(see Lentils, French green)*

Fruit
    The Veggie Queen's Husband's Daily Green
        Smoothie, 40

G

Garbanzo bean flour *(see Chickpea flour)*

Garlic *(see Alliums)*

Garlic powder
    All Purpose Salt-Free Spicy Mix, 89
    Millet, Sunflower Seed, Chili-Garlic Sauce, 225
    Scalloped Turnips Casserole, 54
    Summer Arugula Salad with Lemon Tahini
        Dressing, 6
    Taco Nut "Meat", 230
    Yam Boats with Chickpeas, Bok Choy and
        Cashew Dill Sauce, 9

Ginger *(see Spices, Ginger)*

Gravy
    Fat-Free "Forks Over Knives"-Style Onion
        Mushroom Gravy, 110

Goji berry
    Kale-Apple Slaw with Goji Berry Dressing, 37

Green beans
    Chickpea Curry, 160
    Green Beans with Nut Cream Dressing on
        Minced Tomato Salad, 216
    Leek and Butternut Squash Soup, 105
    Spicy Red Lentil Vegetable Soup, 177

Green onions *(see Alliums)*

Greens *(also see individual names)*
    Black Bean and Greens Quesadillas with
        Smoky Chipotle Cream, 151
    Garlic, Greens, and Tofu with a Twist, 97
    Go-To Winter Medley, 112
    Gutsy Greek Gigantes Beans with Greens,
        Oregano and Mint, 79
    Lemony Lentil and Potato Chowder, 168
    Mediterranean Greens, 34
    Nourishing Stew, 175
    Protein Powerhouse Trifecta, 150
    Rutabaga "Noodles" with Lemon Balsamic
        Tahini Sauce, 50
    Slow Cooker Yellow-Eyed Bean Soup with
        Sweet Potatoes and Greens, 193
    Smoky Sweet Black-Eyed Peas, 159
    Split Pea and Yam Soup, 189

H

Hemp seeds *(see Seeds, Hemp)*

Herbs *(see ingredients below)*

Basil
    8-Minute Split Pea Soup, 187
    Cabbage Lime Salad with Dijon-Lime
        Dressing, 22
    Garden Bruschetta, 65
    Herbed Sunflower Seed Dip or Spread with a
        Fermented "Cheeze" Variation, 228
    Herbed Tofu Dressing, 80
    Herby Italian Dressing, 80
    Pasta with Zesty Lemon White Bean Sauce, 191
    Perfect Pesto Stuffed Mushrooms (raw), 66
    Quick-Stuffed Crimini Mushrooms, 125
    Roasted Cauliflower with Arugula Pesto, 31
    Stuffed Herb Pesto Holiday Appetizers, 67
    Summer Seasoning Blend, 87
    Thai Rice, Snow Pea and Mushroom Salad, 180
    Zesty Broccoli Rabe with Chickpeas and
        Pasta, 16

Bay leaf
    8-Minute Split Pea Soup, 187
    Brazilian Black Bean Stew (Feijoada), 155
    Lentil Coconut Spinach Soup, 170
    Lentil-Leek Soup, 172
    Minted Pea Soup, 179
    M'jeddrah, 174
    Shiitake Mushroom Asparagus Spinach Soup,
        140
    Spicy Red Lentil Vegetable Soup, 177
    Vegan Red Beans and Rice, 167
    Wild Mushroom and Farro Stew, 131

Cilantro
    Asian Bean Dip, 190
    Black Bean and Greens Quesadillas with
        Smoky Chipotle Cream, 151
    Carrots Stir-fried with Mung Sprouts and
        Vegetables, 68
    Cilantro Avocado Dressing, 70
    Falafel Patties, 163
    Fresh Fruit Chutney with Mustard Seeds and
        Cilantro, 109
    Ginger Lime Carrot Soup, 74
    Kale Apply Curry, 86
    Spiced Cauliflower, 72
    Spicy Black Bean Dip, 156

Stuffed Herb Pesto Holiday Appetizers, 67
   Thai Rice, Snow Pea and Mushroom Salad, 180
   Tomatillo Black Bean Salsa, 70
   Trumpet Mushroom and Avocado Ceviche, 144
Dill
   Potato and Watercress Soup with Sorrel
     Cream, 55
Marjoram
   Cream of Brussels Sprouts Soup with Vegan
     Cream Sauce, 17
   Slow Cooker Yellow-Eyed Bean Soup with
     Sweet Potatoes and Greens, 193
   Summer Seasoning Blend, 87
Mint
   Chickpea and Strawberry Summer Salad, 161
   Crunchy Kohlrabi Quinoa Salad, 42
   Gutsy Greek Gigantes Beans with Greens,
     Oregano and Mint, 79
   Lemony Lentil and Potato Chowder, 168
   Minted Pea Soup, 179
   Raw Cauliflower Tabbouleh, 28
   Rutabaga "Noodles" with Lemon Balsamic
     Tahini Sauce, 50
   Summer Seasoning Blend, 87
   Trumpet Mushroom and Avocado Ceviche, 144
Oregano
   8-Minute Split Pea Soup, 187
   All Purpose Salt-Free Spicy Mix, 89
   Black Bean and Greens Quesadillas with
     Smoky Chipotle Cream, 151
   Greek Garbanzo Bean Salad, 164
   Gutsy Greek Gigantes Beans with Greens,
     Oregano and Mint, 79
   Herb and Chile Rub, 90
   Split Pea and Yam Soup, 189
   Stir-Fry Toppings, 14
   Sweet Potato Flatbread, 212
Parsley
   8-Minute Split Pea Soup, 187
   Allium Broth, 95
   All Purpose Salt-Free Spicy Mix, 89
   Arugula and Herb Pesto, 3
   Baked Stuffed Onions, 107
   Chickpea and Strawberry Summer Salad, 161
   Crunchy Kohlrabi Quinoa Salad, 42
   Garlic Herb Aioli, 99
   Greek Garbanzo Bean Salad, 164

Herbed Sesame Crackers, 221
Herbed Sunflower Seed Dip or Spread with a
   Fermented "Cheeze" Variation, 228
Herbed Tofu Dressing, 80
Herby Italian Dressing, 80
Lentil, Mushroom and Walnut Paté, 123
Minted Pea Soup, 179
Mushroom Un–Meatballs, 138
Parsley Pistachio Lime Pesto, 81
Pepita Parsnip Paté, 219
Raw Cauliflower Tabbouleh, 28
Rutabaga "Noodles" with Lemon Balsamic
   Tahini Sauce, 50
Scalloped Turnips Casserole, 54
Stuffed Herb Pesto Holiday Appetizers, 67
Tuscan Soup with a Twist, 192
Watercress-Sage Pesto, 56
Wild Mushroom Ravioli, 142
Rosemary
   8-Minute Split Pea Soup, 187
   All Purpose Salt-Free Spicy Mix, 89
   Balsamic Glazed Herb Roasted Roots with
     Kohlrabi, Rutabaga, Turnip, Chickpea
     Tomato Soup, 162
   Fennel, Carrots and Potatoes, 43
   Grain-Free Just Seeds Crackers, 226
   Red Lentil Soup with Sweet Potatoes and
     Spinach, 176
   Rosemary Mushrooms and Kale, 127
   Slow Cooker Yellow-Eyed Bean Soup with
     Sweet Potatoes and Greens, 193
   Tempeh and Wild Mushroom Stew, 141
   Umami Sun-Dried Tomato and Almond
     Burgers, 202
Sage
   Allium Broth, 95
   All Purpose Salt-Free Spicy Mix, 89
   Pasta with Creamy Cashew Maitake
     Mushroom Sauce, 132
   Watercress-Sage Pesto, 56
Thyme
   Allium Broth, 95
   All Purpose Salt-Free Spicy Mix, 89
   Baby Leeks a la Nicoise, 104
   Balsamic Glazed Herb Roasted Roots with
     Kohlrabi, Rutabaga, Turnip, Fennel, Carrots
     and Potatoes, 43

Braised Green Cabbage, 20
Braised Turnip Greens with Tomatoes and
   Thyme, 52
Herb and Chile Rub, 90
Lentil Coconut Spinach Soup, 170
Lentil, Mushroom and Walnut Paté, 123
Mushroom Thyme Sauce, 83
Roasted Beet Hummus with Thyme, 82
Summer Seasoning Blend, 87
Vegan Red Beans and Rice, 167
Wild Mushroom and Farro Stew, 131
"Herbs and Spices Flavor Profiles", 64
"Herbs and Spices Flavor Families", 64

Herbs and Spices (see ingredients below)
Horseradish
   Barley, White Beans, and Horseradish Sauce, 25
   Horseradish and Cannellini Bean Dip, 36
Hummus
   Hummus, 165
   No-Bean Hummus, 220
   Roasted Beet Hummus with Thyme, 82

I

Ingredient Sources, 244

J

Jalapeno *(see Spices, Chile)*

K

Kaffir lime leaves
   Thai-Inspired Broccoli Slaw, 15
   Thai Rice, Snow Pea and Mushroom Salad, 180
Kale
   Easy Salsa Supper, 157
   Hail to the Kale Salad, 38
   Immune Power Soup, 137
   Kale Apple Almond Milk, 199
   Kale-Apple Slaw with Goji Berry Dressing, 37
   Kale and Spring Pea Mash-up, 182
   Kale Apply Curry, 86
   Kale Cabbage Coleslaw with Sunflower Seed
      Spicy Thai Dressing, 227
   Kid's Kale, 39
   Protein Powerhouse Trifecta, 150
   The Veggie Queen's Husband's Daily Green
      Smoothie, 40
   The Veggie Queen's Raw Kale Salad, 41

Kohlrabi
   Crunchy Kohlrabi Quinoa Salad, 42
   Lentil Coconut Spinach Soup, 170
Kumquats
   Mustard Greens, Snow Peas, Green Garlic and
      Kumquats Spring Slaw, 46

L

Leek *(see Alliums)*

Legumes *(see Pulses: Beans, Peas, Lentils)*

Lemon juice or zest
   Chickpea and Strawberry Summer Salad, 161
   Collard Greens Wrapped Rolls with Spiced
      Quinoa Filling, 33
   Creamy Caesar Salad Dressing, 96
   Crunchy Kohlrabi Quinoa Salad, 42
   Curried Lentils and Spinach, 169
   Daikon Radish Rawvioli with Creamy Nut
      Filling, 48
   Falafel Patties, 163
   French Green Lentil Salad with Asparagus and
      Pine Nuts, 173
   Garlic Herb Aioli, 99
   Garlic, Greens, and Tofu with a Twist, 97
   Greek Garbanzo Bean Salad, 164
   Herbed Sesame Crackers, 221
   Herbed Sunflower Seed Dip or Spread with a
      Fermented "Cheeze" Variation, 228
   Hummus, 165
   Summer Seasoning Blend, 87
   Kale and Spring Pea Mash-up, 182
   Kid's Kale, 39
   Lemon Scented Spinach Spread, 103
   Lemony Lentil and Potato Chowder, 168
   Macadamia Yellow Cheese, 214
   Pasta with Zesty Lemon White Bean Sauce, 191
   Perfect Pesto Stuffed Mushrooms (raw), 66
   Potato and Watercress Soup with Sorrel
      Cream, 55
   Raw Cauliflower Tabbouleh, 28
   Roasted Cauliflower with Arugula Pesto, 31
   Romaine Burritos, 201
   Shiitake Mushroom Asparagus Spinach
      Soup, 140
   Stuffed Herb Pesto Holiday Appetizers, 67
   Sweet Potato Flatbread, 212
   Wonder Spread, 207

Lemongrass
   Thai-Inspired Broccoli Slaw, 15
   Thai Rice, Snow Pea and Mushroom Salad, 180

Lentils: Pulses *(see ingredients below)*

 Brown or Green
   Curried Lentils and Spinach, 169
   Lentil Coconut Spinach Soup, 170
   Lentil-Leek Soup, 172
   Lentil, Mushroom and Walnut Paté, 123
   Stir-Fry Toppings, 14

 French green
   French Green Lentil Salad with Asparagus and
      Pine Nuts, 173
   Rainbow Sprout Salad, 178

 Red
   Lemony Lentil and Potato Chowder, 168
   M'jeddrah, 174
   Nourishing Stew, 175
   Quick Lentil and Eggplant Curry, 85
   Red Lentil Soup with Sweet Potatoes and
      Spinach, 176
   Root Veggies Paté, 49
   Spicy Red Lentil Vegetable Soup, 177

Lettuce
   Minted Pea Soup, 179
   Romaine Burritos, 201

Lime juice
   Black Bean and Greens Quesadillas with
      Smoky Chipotle Cream, 151
   Cabbage Lime Salad with Dijon-Lime
      Dressing, 22
   Cilantro Avocado Dressing, 70
   Fresh Fruit Chutney with Mustard Seeds and
      Cilantro, 109
   Hail to the Kale Salad, 38
   Kale Cabbage Coleslaw with Sunflower Seed
      Spicy Thai Dressing, 227
   Kidney Bean Salad with Chili-Lime Dressing, 166
   Lentil Coconut Spinach Soup, 170
   Lime and Ginger Fruit Salad, 77
   Nourishing Stew, 175
   Parsley Pistachio Lime Pesto, 81
   Red Almond Cheese, 200
   Roasted Beet Hummus with Thyme, 82
   Root Veggies Paté, 49
   Spicy Black Bean Dip, 156
   Spicy Peanut Citrus Sauce, 217

   Summer Arugula Salad with Lemon Tahini
      Dressing, 6
   Thai-Inspired Broccoli Slaw, 15
   Thai Rice, Snow Pea and Mushroom Salad, 180
   Tomatillo Black Bean Salsa, 70
   Trumpet Mushroom and Avocado Ceviche, 144

Lime, Kaffir *(see Kaffir lime)*

"Lovely Legumes: Full of Beans", 148

M

Maitake mushroom *(see Mushrooms)*

Mango
   Mango, Daikon, and Avocado Spring Rolls, 49

Maple syrup
   Balsamic Glazed Herb Roasted Roots with
      Kohlrabi, Rutabaga, Turnip, Fennel, Carrots
      and Potatoes, 43
   Cabbage and Red Apple Slaw, 21
   Creamy House Dressing, 205
   Fresh Fruit Chutney with Mustard Seeds and
      Cilantro, 109
   Ginger-Pineapple Pudding, 76
   Jill's Mustard Blend, 78
   Spicy Peanut Citrus Sauce, 217
   Wonder Spread, 207

Marjoram *(see Herbs)*

Matcha (green tea) powder
   Raw Almond Matcha Cakes, 199

Millet
   Millet, Sunflower Seed, Chili-Garlic Sauce, 225

Milk, nondairy *(see Nondairy milk)*

Mint *(see Herbs)*

Miso
   Asian Bean Dip, 190
   Creamy Ginger-Hemp Dressing, 213
   Garlic Herb Aioli, 99
   Immune Power Soup, 137
   Miso Vegetable Soup, 185
   Pepita Parsnip Paté, 219
   Perfect Pesto Stuffed Mushrooms (raw), 66
   Protein Powerhouse Trifecta, 150
   Rainbow Sprout Salad, 178
   Sesame Bok Choy Shiitake Stir Fry, 7
   Super Spring Salad with Zesty Orange
      Dressing, 77
   Tempeh and Wild Mushroom Stew, 141

The Veggie Queen's Raw Kale Salad, 41
Wild Mushroom Ravioli, 142
Wonder Spread, 207

Mushrooms *(see ingredients below)*

"A Word about the Mushrooms", 110

Fat-Free "Forks Over Knives"-Style Onion
Mushroom Gravy, 110

Crimini
Brazilian Black Bean Stew (Feijoada), 155
Coconut-Chickpea Crepes with Smoky Herbed
Mushrooms, 122
Lentil, Mushroom and Walnut Paté, 123
Mushroom Un–Meatballs, 138
Perfect Pesto Stuffed Mushrooms (raw), 66
Quick-Stuffed Crimini Mushrooms, 125
Rich Mushroom Gravy, 126
Rosemary Mushrooms and Kale, 127
Tatsoi with Bok Choy and Mushrooms, 51
Tempeh and Wild Mushroom Stew, 141
Veggie Mushroom Burgers, 129
Wild Mushroom and Farro Stew, 131

Dried wild mixed
Fat-Free "Forks Over Knives"-Style Onion
Mushroom Gravy, 110
Mushroom Un–Meatballs, 138
Tempeh and Wild Mushroom Stew, 141

Maitake
Pasta with Creamy Cashew Maitake
Mushroom Sauce, 132
Roasted Maitake, 133

Oyster
Oyster Mushroom, Asparagus and Tofu Stir
Fry, 134

Portabello
Grilled Mushroom and Spring Onion Salad
with Miso Tahini Dressing, 135
Stir-Fry Toppings, 14

Reishi, 120
Immune Broth, 136

Shiitake
Immune Broth, 136
Immune Power Soup, 137
Mushroom Un–Meatballs, 138
Sesame Bok Choy Shiitake Stir Fry, 7
Simple Shiitake and Broccoli (Mock) Stir-Fry, 139
Shiitake Mushroom Asparagus Spinach Soup, 140

Tempeh and Wild Mushroom Stew, 141
Thai Rice, Snow Pea and Mushroom Salad, 180
Wild Mushroom and Farro Stew, 131
Wild Mushroom Ravioli, 142

Trumpet
Smoked Trumpet Mushroom Potato Soup, 143
Trumpet Mushroom and Avocado Ceviche, 144

Turkey Tail
Immune Broth, 136

White button
Coconut-Chickpea Crepes with Smoky Herbed
Mushrooms, 122
Cream of Brussels Sprouts Soup with Vegan
Cream Sauce, 17
Kale and Spring Pea Mash-up, 182
Mushroom Oat Burgers, 145
Tuscan Soup with a Twist, 192

Mustard *(prepared, Dijon and other)*
Cabbage and Red Apple Slaw, 21
Cabbage Lime Salad with Dijon-Lime
Dressing, 22
Creamy Caesar Salad Dressing, 96
Creamy House Dressing, 205
Garlic Herb Aioli, 99
Garlicky Lemon Spinach Salad with Sunflower
Seeds, Olives and Sprouted Beans, 100
Lemon Scented Spinach Spread, 103
Rainbow Sprout Salad, 178

Mustard greens
Bok Choy, Green Garlic and Greens with
Sweet Ginger Sauce, 8
Mustard Greens and Gumbo, 44
Mustard Greens, Snow Peas, Green Garlic and
Kumquats Spring Slaw, 46

Mustard powder
Jill's Mustard Blend, 78

Mustard seeds *(see Spices)*

N

Nondairy cheese *(see Cheese, nondairy)*

Nondairy Milk
Banana Nut Chia Pudding, 209
Black Bean Peanut Butter Brownies, 154
Cashew Almond Date Milk, 205
Hemp Seed Chocolate Mylk, 213
Fat-Free "Forks Over Knives"-Style Onion
Mushroom Gravy, 110

Ginger Lime Carrot Soup, 74
   Ginger-Pineapple Pudding, 76
   Kale Apple Almond Milk, 199
   Leek and Potato Soup, 106
   Minted Pea Soup, 179
   Pasta with Zesty Lemon White Bean Sauce, 191
   Pumpkin Seed and Chocolate Chip Oatmeal
      Breakfast Bars, 218
   Roasted Stuffed Onions with Carrot-Potato
      Purée, 113
   Scalloped Turnips Casserole, 54
   Shiitake Mushroom Asparagus Spinach Soup,
      140

Nutmeg *(see Spices)*

Nutritional yeast
   All Purpose Salt-Free Spicy Mix, 89
   Baked Stuffed Onions, 107
   Collard Green and Quinoa Taco or Burrito
      Filling, 32
   Fat-Free "Forks Over Knives"-Style Onion
      Mushroom Gravy, 110
   Garlic Herb Aioli, 99
   Horseradish and Cannellini Bean Dip, 36
   Kale and Spring Pea Mash-up, 182
   Lemon-Pepper Arugula Pizza with White Bean
      Basil Sauce, 4
   Rich Mushroom Gravy, 126
   Scalloped Turnips Casserole, 54
   Sweet Watercress Smoothie, 57
   Wonder Spread, 207

Nuts *(see ingredients below)*

  Spiced Nuts, 91

  Almonds
    Banana Nut Chia Pudding, 209
    Cashew Almond Date Milk, 205
    Creamy Caesar Salad Dressing, 96
    Hazelnut Sesame Bars, 220
    Hail to the Kale Salad, 38
    Kale Apple Almond Milk, 199
    Raw Almond Matcha Cakes, 199
    Red Almond Cheese, 200
    Romaine Burritos, 201
    The Veggie Queen's Husband's Daily Green
       Smoothie, 40
    Umami Sun-Dried Tomato and Almond
       Burgers, 202

Brazil
   High-Fiber Blueberry, Pear, and Spinach
      Smoothie with Brazil Nuts, 203

Cashews
   Banana Nut Chia Pudding, 209
   Cashew Almond Date Milk, 205
   Cream of Brussels Sprouts Soup with Vegan
      Cream Sauce, 17
   Creamy Cashew Almond Custard, 204
   Creamy House Dressing, 205
   Creamy Southern Soup Beans, 183
   Daikon Radish Rawvioli with Creamy Nut
      Filling, 48
   Pasta with Creamy Cashew Maitake
      Mushroom Sauce, 132
   Raw Cashew and Tahini Dressing, 206
   Raw Chia Seed Pudding with Cinnamon, 211
   Wonder Spread, 207
   Spiced Cauliflower, 72
   Tofu and Snow Pea Stir Fry Salad, 101
   Yam Boats with Chickpeas, Bok Choy and
      Cashew Dill Sauce, 9

Hazelnuts (filberts)
   Hazelnut Sesame Bars, 220

Macadamia
   Macadamia Yellow Cheese, 214

Peanuts
   Decadent Chocolate Peanut Butter Truffles, 215
   Green Beans with Nut Cream Dressing on
      Minced Tomato Salad, 216
   Spicy Peanut Citrus Sauce, 217
   Thai Rice, Snow Pea and Mushroom Salad, 180

Pine Nuts
   Arugula and Herb Pesto, 3
   Collard Greens Wrapped Rolls with Spiced
      Quinoa Filling, 33
   French Green Lentil Salad with Asparagus and
      Pine Nuts, 173
   Perfect Pesto Stuffed Mushrooms (raw), 66
   Raw Cauliflower Tabbouleh, 28
   Stuffed Herb Pesto Holiday Appetizers, 67

Pistachio
   Parsley Pistachio Lime Pesto, 81

Walnuts
   Baked Stuffed Onions, 107
   Cherry-Chocolate Walnut Truffles, 229

Macadamia Yellow Cheese, 214
Quick-Stuffed Crimini Mushrooms, 125
Raw Cinnamon Rolls, 230
Roasted Cauliflower with Arugula Pesto, 31
Taco Nut "Meat", 230

O

Oats
Lentil, Mushroom and Walnut Paté, 123
Mushroom Oat Burgers, 145
Mushroom Un–Meatballs, 138
Overnight Muesli, 210
Pumpkin Seed and Chocolate Chip Oatmeal
Breakfast Bars, 218
Veggie Mushroom Burgers, 129

Oil
"The Great Oil Debate In Which I Refuse to
Participate", 58

Olives
Baked Stuffed Onions, 107
Garden Bruschetta, 65
Garlicky Lemon Spinach Salad with
Sunflower Seeds, Olives and Sprouted
Beans, 100
Greek Garbanzo Bean Salad, 164
Mediterranean Greens, 34
Raw Cauliflower Tabbouleh, 28
Rutabaga "Noodles" with Lemon Balsamic
Tahini Sauce, 50

Onion (see Alliums)

Onion powder
All Purpose Salt-Free Spicy Mix, 89
Herb and Chile Rub, 90
Shangri-La Soup, 5
Taco Nut "Meat", 230

Orange, juice and zest
Creamy Ginger-Hemp Dressing, 213
Mustard Greens, Snow Peas, Green Garlic
and Kumquats Spring Slaw, 46
Rainbow Sprout Salad, 178
Spicy Peanut Citrus Sauce, 217
Super Spring Salad with Zesty Orange
Dressing, 77

Oregano (see Herbs)

Oyster Mushroom (see Mushrooms)

P

Parsley (see Herbs)

Parsnip
Leek and Butternut Squash Soup, 105
Pepita Parsnip Paté, 219
Roasted Beet Hummus with Thyme, 82

Pasta
Greek Garbanzo Bean Salad, 164
Pasta with Creamy Cashew Maitake
Mushroom Sauce, 132
Pasta with Zesty Lemon White Bean Sauce, 191
Zesty Broccoli Rabe with Chickpeas and
Pasta, 16

Paté
Lentil, Mushroom and Walnut Paté, 123
Pepita Parsnip Paté, 219
Root Veggies Paté, 49

Peaches
Lime and Ginger Fruit Salad, 77

Peanuts (see Nuts, Peanut)

Peanut butter
Asian Bean Dip, 190
Black Bean Peanut Butter Brownies, 154
Decadent Chocolate Peanut Butter Truffles, 215
Spicy Peanut Citrus Sauce, 217
Thai-Inspired Broccoli Slaw, 15

Pear
High-Fiber Blueberry, Pear, and Spinach
Smoothie with Brazil Nuts, 203

Peas, Black-Eyed
Easy Salsa Supper, 157
Fresh Shelling Beans and Summer Vegetables, 158
Smoky Sweet Black-Eyed Peas, 159

Peas, English
Kale and Spring Pea Mash-up, 182
Minted Pea Soup, 179
Nourishing Stew, 175

Peas, Snow or Sugar Snap
Crunchy Kohlrabi Quinoa Salad, 42
Mustard Greens, Snow Peas, Green Garlic and
Kumquats Spring Slaw, 46
Thai Rice, Snow Pea and Mushroom Salad, 180
Tofu and Snow Pea Stir Fry Salad, 101

Peas, Split Green
Chef AJ's 8 Minute Split Pea Soup, 187

Split Pea and Yam Soup, 189

Pepper, Black *(also see Spices)*
All Purpose Salt-Free Spicy Mix, 89
Cocoa Spice Powder, 89

Peppers, sweet
Black Bean Collard Wraps, 153
Cabbage Lime Salad with Dijon-Lime Dressing, 22
Fennel with Broccoli, Zucchini and Peppers, 12
Fresh Shelling Beans and Summer Vegetables, 158
Moroccan Vegetable Tagine, 53
Mushroom Oat Burgers, 145
Mustard Greens and Gumbo, 44
Kale Cabbage Coleslaw with Sunflower Seed Spicy Thai Dressing, 227
Kidney Bean Salad with Chili-Lime Dressing, 166
Quick Lentil and Eggplant Curry, 85
Red Almond Cheese, 200
Stir-Fry Toppings, 14
Smoky Sweet Black-Eyed Peas, 159
Spicy Red Lentil Vegetable Soup, 177
Summer Arugula Salad with Lemon Tahini Dressing, 6
Thai Rice, Snow Pea and Mushroom Salad, 180
Trumpet Mushroom and Avocado Ceviche, 144

Peppers, hot *(see Chile Peppers)*

Pesto
Arugula and Herb Pesto, 3
Parsley Pistachio Lime Pesto, 81
Roasted Cauliflower with Arugula Pesto, 31
Stuffed Herb Pesto Holiday Appetizers, 67
Watercress-Sage Pesto, 56

Pine Nuts *(see Nuts, Pine)*

Pineapple and juice
Ginger-Pineapple Pudding, 76
Sweet Watercress Smoothie, 57

Pinto Beans *(see Beans, Pinto)*

Pistachio *(see Nuts, Pistachio)*

Pizza
Lemon-Pepper Arugula Pizza with White Bean Basil Sauce, 4
"Maizing" Brassica Pizza, 223
Really Reubenesque Revisited Pizza, 23

Pizza Dough
Pumpernickel or Rye Dough, 23

Wheat and Black Bean Dough, 224

Pomegranate
Kale Cabbage Coleslaw with Sunflower Seed Spicy Thai Dressing, 227

Portabello Mushroom *(see Mushrooms)*

Potato
8-Minute Split Pea Soup, 187
Balsamic Glazed Herb Roasted Roots with Kohlrabi, Rutabaga, Turnip, Fennel, Carrots and Potatoes, 43
Chickpea Curry, 160
Creamy Dreamy Broccoli Soup, 11
Curried White and Sweet Potato Pancakes with Fresh Fruit Chutney, 108
Garlic, Greens, and Tofu with a Twist, 97
Lemony Lentil and Potato Chowder, 168
Minted Pea Soup, 179
Potato and Watercress Soup with Sorrel Cream, 55
Quick Lentil and Eggplant Curry, 85
Roasted Stuffed Onions with Carrot-Potato Purée, 113
Smoked Trumpet Mushroom Potato Soup, 143
Split Pea and Yam Soup, 189
Veggie Mushroom Burgers, 129

Potsticker or wonton wrappers
Wild Mushroom Ravioli, 142

Preserves, apricot or orange marmalade
Garlic, Greens, and Tofu with a Twist, 97

Pressure cooker
"The Pressure Cooker and Pulses Can Save Your Life or at Least Your Time", 188

Pressure cooker recipes
8-Minute Split Pea Soup, 187
Braised Cabbage with Cumin, 73
Lentil Coconut Spinach Soup, 170
Minted Pea Soup, 179
Spicy Red Lentil Vegetable Soup, 177

Pulses *(see Beans, Lentils or Peas)*

Q

Quinoa
Baked Stuffed Onions, 107
Collard Green and Quinoa Taco or Burrito Filling, 32

Collard Greens Wrapped Rolls with Spiced
  Quinoa Filling, 33
Easy Salsa Supper, 157
Go-To Winter Medley, 112
Nourishing Stew, 175
Pinto Bean Quinoa Burgers, 184
Protein Powerhouse Trifecta, 150
Umami Sun-Dried Tomato and Almond
  Burgers, 202

R

Radish
  Cinnamon Roasted Radishes, 47
  Crunchy Kohlrabi Quinoa Salad, 42
  Daikon Radish Rawvioli with Creamy Nut
    Filling, 48
  Mango, Daikon, and Avocado Spring Rolls, 49
  Rice and Veggie Sushi Salad, 186

Raisins
  Banana Nut Chia Pudding, 209
  Black Bean Peanut Butter Brownies, 154
  Collard Greens Wrapped Rolls with Spiced
    Quinoa Filling, 33
  Kale Apply Curry, 86
  Mediterranean Greens, 34
  Raw Cinnamon Rolls, 230

Rice, Brown and Other
  Black Bean Collard Wraps, 153
  Leek and Butternut Squash Soup, 105
  M'jeddrah, 174
  Mushroom Oat Burgers, 145
  Mustard Greens and Gumbo, 44
  Rice and Veggie Sushi Salad, 186
  Thai Rice, Snow Pea and Mushroom Salad, 180
  Veggie Mushroom Burgers, 129

Rice noodles
  Thai Bangkok Noodles, 115

Romaine lettuce (see Lettuce)

Romanesco broccoli (see Broccoli, Romanesco)

Rosemary (see Herbs)

Rutabaga
  Balsamic Glazed Herb Roasted Roots with
    Kohlrabi, Rutabaga, Turnip, Fennel, Carrots
    and Potatoes, 43
  Root Veggies Paté, 49
  Rutabaga "Noodles" with Lemon Balsamic
    Tahini Sauce, 50

S

Sage (see Herbs)

Sake
  Trumpet Mushroom and Avocado Ceviche, 144

Salad dressing
  Chili-Lime Dressing, 166
  Cilantro Avocado Dressing, 70
  Creamy Caesar Salad Dressing, 96
  Creamy Ginger-Hemp Dressing, 213
  Creamy House Dressing, 205
  Dijon-Lime Dressing, 22
  Goji Berry Dressing, 37
  Herbed Tofu Dressing, 80
  Herby Italian Dressing, 80
  Lemon Tahini Dressing, 6
  Miso Tahini Dressing, 135
  Raw Cashew and Tahini Dressing, 206
  Zesty Orange Dressing, 77

Salads
  Cabbage Lime Salad with Dijon-Lime
    Dressing, 22
  Chickpea and Strawberry Summer Salad, 161
  Crunchy Kohlrabi Quinoa Salad, 42
  Garlic Sesame Broccoli Salad, 99
  Garlicky Lemon Spinach Salad with Sunflower
    Seeds, Olives and Sprouted Beans, 100
  Greek Garbanzo Bean Salad, 164
  Grilled Mushroom and Spring Onion Salad
    with Miso Tahini Dressing, 135
  Hail to the Kale Salad, 38
  Kale-Apple Slaw with Goji Berry Dressing, 37
  Kidney Bean Salad with Chili-Lime Dressing, 166
  Raw Cauliflower Tabbouleh, 28
  Rice and Veggie Sushi Salad, 186
  Smoky Sweet Black-Eyed Peas, 159
  Summer Arugula Salad with Lemon Tahini
    Dressing, 6
  Super Spring Salad with Zesty Orange
    Dressing, 77
  Thai Rice, Snow Pea and Mushroom Salad, 180
  The Veggie Queen's Raw Kale Salad, 41
  Tofu and Snow Pea Stir Fry Salad, 101

Salsa
  Easy Salsa Supper, 157

Sauces
  Barley, White Beans, and Horseradish Sauce, 25
  Cashew Dill Sauce, 9

Creamy Cashew Maitake Mushroom Sauce, 132
Lemon Balsamic Tahini Sauce, 50
Millet, Sunflower Seeds, and Chili-Garlic
 Sauce, 225
Mushroom Thyme Sauce, 83
Romanesco Broccoli Sauce, 13
Smoky Chipotle Cream, 151
Spicy Peanut Citrus Sauce, 217
Thousand Islands Dressing Sauce, 25
Vegan Cream Sauce, 17
White Bean Basil Sauce, 4

Sea Vegetables/Seaweed

Gomasio: Seaweed, Seeds and Salt Sprinkle, 222
Kale Cabbage Coleslaw with Sunflower Seed
 Spicy Thai Dressing, 227

Agar agar
 Blueberry Gel, 71
 Creamy Cashew Almond Custard, 204
 Ginger-Pineapple Pudding, 76
Dulse
 Gomasio: Seaweed, Seeds and Salt Sprinkle, 222
Kombu
 Immune Broth, 136
 Roasted Beet Hummus with Thyme, 82
Nori
 Rice and Veggie Sushi Salad, 186
 Trumpet Mushroom and Avocado Ceviche, 144
Wakame
 Miso Vegetable Soup, 185

Seeds (see ingredients below)

Chia
 Banana Nut Chia Pudding, 209
 Dr. Shiroko Sokitch's Favorite Breakfast, 208
 Overnight Muesli, 210
 Raw Chia Seed Pudding with Cinnamon, 211
 Sweet Watercress Smoothie, 57
 The Veggie Queen's Husband's Daily Green
  Smoothie, 40
Flax
 Gomasio: Seaweed, Seeds and Salt Sprinkle, 222
 Grain-Free Just Seeds Crackers, 226
 Herbed Sesame Crackers, 221
 Mushroom Oat Burgers, 145
 Sweet Potato Flatbread, 212
 Sweet Watercress Smoothie, 57
 Veggie Mushroom Burgers, 129

Hemp
 Creamy Ginger-Hemp Dressing, 213
 Dr. Shiroko Sokitch's Favorite Breakfast, 208
 Grain-Free Just Seeds Crackers, 226
 Hemp Seed Chocolate Mylk, 213
 Pinto Bean Quinoa Burgers, 184
Pumpkin
 Grain-Free Just Seeds Crackers, 226
 Pumpkin Seed and Chocolate Chip Oatmeal
  Breakfast Bars, 218
 Pepita Parsnip Paté, 219
Sesame
 Bok Choy, Green Garlic and Greens with
  Sweet Ginger Sauce, 8
 Garlic Sesame Broccoli Salad, 99
 Gingered Cucumber Salad, 75
 Gomasio: Seaweed, Seeds and Salt Sprinkle, 222
 Grain-Free Just Seeds Crackers, 226
 Hazelnut Sesame Bars, 220
 Herbed Sesame Crackers, 221
 No-Bean Hummus, 220
 Rice and Veggie Sushi Salad, 186
 Seaweed, Seeds and Salt Sprinkle, 222
 Sesame Bok Choy Shiitake Stir Fry, 7
Sunflower
 Garlicky Lemon Spinach Salad with Sunflower
  Seeds, Olives and Sprouted Beans, 100
 Grain-Free Just Seeds Crackers, 226
 Herbed Sunflower Seed Dip or Spread with a
  Fermented "Cheeze" Variation, 228
 Kale Cabbage Coleslaw with Sunflower Seed
  Millet, Sunflower Seeds, and Chili-Garlic
  Sauce, 225
 Protein Powerhouse Trifecta, 150
 Rainbow Sprout Salad, 178
 Spicy Thai Dressing, 227
 Watercress-Sage Pesto, 56

Shallots (see Alliums)

Shiitake Mushrooms (see Mushrooms)

Slaw
 Cabbage and Red Apple Slaw, 21
 Kale Cabbage Coleslaw with Sunflower Seed
  Spicy Thai Dressing, 227
 Mustard Greens, Snow Peas, Green Garlic and
  Kumquats Spring Slaw, 46
 Thai-Inspired Broccoli Slaw, 15

Slow Cooker recipes
Asian-Adzuki Bean Crockpot Chili, 149
Slow Cooker Yellow-Eyed Bean Soup with
Sweet Potatoes and Greens, 193
Smoothie
High-Fiber Blueberry, Pear, and Spinach
Smoothie with Brazil Nuts, 203
Sweet Watercress Smoothie, 57
The Veggie Queen's Husband's Daily Green
Smoothie, 40
Snow Peas *(see Peas, Snow)*
Sorrel
Potato and Watercress Soup with Sorrel
Cream, 55
Soup
Chickpea Tomato Soup, 162
Cream of Brussels Sprouts Soup with Vegan
Cream Sauce, 17
Creamy Dreamy Broccoli Soup, 11
Immune Broth, 136
Immune Power Soup, 137
Ginger Lime Carrot Soup, 74
Leek and Potato Soup, 106
Lemony Lentil and Potato Chowder, 168
Lentil Coconut Spinach Soup, 170
Lentil-Leek Soup, 172
Minted Pea Soup, 179
Miso Vegetable Soup, 185
Potato and Watercress Soup with Sorrel
Cream, 55
Red Lentil Soup with Sweet Potatoes and
Spinach, 176
Shangri-La Soup, 5
Shiitake Mushroom Asparagus Spinach Soup, 140
Smoked Trumpet Mushroom Potato Soup, 143
Spicy Red Lentil Vegetable Soup, 177
Split Pea and Yam Soup, 189
Tuscan Soup with a Twist, 192
Truffled Celeriac Soup, 121
Soybeans, green, edamame *(see Beans, Soybeans)*

Spices *(see ingredients below)*
Allspice
Vegan Red Beans and Rice, 167
Asafoetida (hing)
Carrots Stir-fried with Mung Sprouts and
Vegetables, 68

Fall Seasoning Blend, 88
Spicy Red Lentil Vegetable Soup, 177
Caraway
Really Reubenesque Revisited Pizza, 23
Cardamom
Spiced Cauliflower, 68
Winter Seasoning Blend, 88
Cayenne
Carrots Stir-fried with Mung Sprouts and
Vegetables, 68
Chickpea Curry, 160
Cocoa-Spice Roasted Squash, 69
Garlic Herb Aioli, 99
Ginger Lime Carrot Soup, 74
Herb and Chile Rub, 90
Herbed Sesame Crackers, 221
Hummus, 165
Lemony Lentil and Potato Chowder, 168
Spiced Cauliflower, 72
Spiced Nuts, 91
Spicy Black Bean Dip, 156
Spring Seasoning Blend, 88
Celery seed
Chef AJ's 8 Minute Split Pea Soup, 187
All Purpose Salt-Free Spicy Mix, 89
Split Pea and Yam Soup, 189
Spring Seasoning Blend, 88
Chiles/Chili Powder
Black Bean and Sweet Potato Hash, 152
Black Bean Collard Wraps, 153
Cocoa-Spice Roasted Squash, 69
Collard Green and Quinoa Taco or Burrito
Filling, 32
Fresh Shelling Beans and Summer Vegetables,
158
Herb and Chile Rub, 90
Immune Broth, 136
Kidney Bean Salad with Chili-Lime Dressing, 166
Smoky Sweet Black-Eyed Peas, 159
Spicy Black Bean Dip, 156
Thai Bangkok Noodles, 115
Thai Rice, Snow Pea and Mushroom Salad, 180
Chipotle powder
Black Bean and Greens Quesadillas with
Smoky Chipotle Cream, 151
Chipotle Cauliflower Mashers, 27
Cocoa Spice Powder, 89

Spiced Nuts, 91
Smoky Collard Greens, 35
Cinnamon
  Blueberry Gel, 71
  Chickpea Curry, 160
  Cocoa Spice Powder, 89
  Collard Greens Wrapped Rolls with Spiced
    Pumpkin Seed and Chocolate Chip Oatmeal
  Breakfast Bars, 218
  Quinoa Filling, 33
  Raw Chia Seed Pudding with Cinnamon, 211
  Raw Cinnamon Rolls, 230
  Spiced Cauliflower, 72
  Spicy Red Lentil Vegetable Soup, 177
  Winter Seasoning Blend, 88
Cloves
  Chickpea Curry, 160
  Spiced Cauliflower, 72
  Winter Seasoning Blend, 88
Coriander
  Chickpea Curry, 160
  Fall Seasoning Blend, 88
  Herb and Chile Rub, 90
  Herbed Sesame Crackers, 221
  Romaine Burritos, 201
  Spiced Cauliflower, 72
  Spicy Red Lentil Vegetable Soup, 177
  Spring Seasoning Blend, 88
  Taco Nut "Meat", 230
Cumin
  Braised Cabbage with Cumin, 73
  Cocoa Spice Powder, 89
  Curried Lentils and Spinach, 169
  Falafel Patties, 163
  Fall Seasoning Blend, 88
  Fresh Shelling Beans and Summer Vegetables,
    158
  Herb and Chile Rub, 90
  Herbed Sesame Crackers, 221
  Hummus, 165
  Kidney Bean Salad with Chili-Lime Dressing, 166
  M'jeddrah, 174
  Nourishing Stew, 175
  Roasted Cauliflower and Chickpea Curry, 29
  Romaine Burritos, 201
  Spiced Cauliflower, 72
  Spicy Black Bean Dip, 156

Split Pea and Yam Soup, 189
Taco Nut "Meat", 230
Tomatillo Black Bean Salsa, 70
Trumpet Mushroom and Avocado Ceviche, 144
Fennel seeds
  Fall Seasoning Blend, 88
  Spicy Red Lentil Vegetable Soup, 177
Fenugreek seed
  Spring Seasoning Blend, 88
Ginger
  Asian Bean Dip, 190
  Bok Choy Ginger Dizzle, 7
  Bok Choy, Green Garlic and Greens with
    Sweet Ginger Sauce, 8
  Broccoli with Turmeric, Ginger and Garlic, 84
  Creamy Ginger-Hemp Dressing, 213
  Curried Lentils and Spinach, 169
  Fall Seasoning Blend, 88
  Ginger Lime Carrot Soup, 74
  Gingered Cucumber Salad, 75
  Ginger-Pineapple Pudding, 76
  Hail to the Kale Salad, 38
  Immune Broth, 136
  Immune Power Soup, 137
  Kale Cabbage Coleslaw with Sunflower Seed
    Spicy Thai Dressing, 227
  Lime and Ginger Fruit Salad, 77
  Nourishing Stew, 175
  Roasted Cauliflower and Chickpea Curry, 29
  Spring Seasoning Blend, 88
  Spicy Red Lentil Vegetable Soup, 177
  Super Spring Salad with Zesty Orange
    Dressing, 77
  Tatsoi with Bok Choy and Mushrooms, 51
  Thai Rice, Snow Pea and Mushroom Salad, 180
  Tofu and Snow Pea Stir Fry Salad, 101
Mustard seed
  Carrots Stir-fried with Mung Sprouts and
    Vegetables, 68
  Fresh Fruit Chutney with Mustard Seeds and
    Cilantro, 109
  Jill's Mustard Blend, 78
  Roasted Cauliflower and Chickpea Curry, 29
  Spring Seasoning Blend, 88
Nutmeg
  Pumpkin Seed and Chocolate Chip Oatmeal
  Breakfast Bars, 218

Truffled Celeriac Soup, 121

Paprika
All Purpose Salt-Free Spicy Mix, 89
Cocoa-Spice Roasted Squash, 69
Herbed Sesame Crackers, 221
Romaine Burritos, 201
Taco Nut "Meat", 230

Paprika, smoked
Chef AJ's 8 Minute Split Pea Soup, 187
Coconut-Chickpea Crepes with Smoky Herbed Mushrooms, 122
Collard Green and Quinoa Taco or Burrito Filling, 32
No-Bean Hummus, 220
Slow Cooker Yellow-Eyed Bean Soup with Sweet Potatoes and Greens, 193
Smoked Trumpet Mushroom Potato Soup, 143
Smoky Sweet Black-Eyed Peas, 159
Taco Nut "Meat", 230
Vegan Red Beans and Rice, 167

Peppercorns
Winter Seasoning Blend, 88

Star Anise
Winter Seasoning Blend, 88

Turmeric
Broccoli with Turmeric, Ginger and Garlic, 84
Fall Seasoning Blend, 88
Carrots Stir-fried with Mung Sprouts and Vegetables, 68
Kale and Spring Pea Mash-up, 182
Nourishing Stew, 175
Roasted Turmeric Brussels Sprouts with Hemp Seeds on Arugula, 19
Spicy Red Lentil Vegetable Soup, 177
Spring Seasoning Blend, 88

Spice Blends
All Purpose Salt-Free Spicy Mix, 89
Cocoa Spice Powder, 89
Herb and Chile Rub, 90
Roasted Cauliflower and Chickpea Curry, 29
Seasonal Spice Blends, 87

Spinach
Baked Stuffed Onions, 107
Cream of Brussels Sprouts Soup with Vegan Cream Sauce, 17
Curried Lentils and Spinach, 169
Garlicky Lemon Spinach Salad with Sunflower Seeds, Olives and Sprouted Beans, 100
Gutsy Greek Gigantes Beans with Greens, Oregano and Mint, 79
High-Fiber Blueberry, Pear, and Spinach Lemon Scented Spinach Spread, 103
Red Lentil Soup with Sweet Potatoes and Spinach, 176
Shiitake Mushroom Asparagus Spinach Soup, 140
Smoothie with Brazil Nuts, 203
Thai Bangkok Noodles, 115

Sprouts
Carrots Stir-fried with Mung Sprouts and Vegetables, 68
Garlicky Lemon Spinach Salad with Sunflower Seeds, Olives and Sprouted Beans, 100
Rice and Veggie Sushi Salad, 186
Thai Bangkok Noodles, 115

Squash, Summer
Bok Choy Ginger Dizzle, 7
Fennel with Broccoli, Zucchini and Peppers, 12
No-Bean Hummus, 220
Nourishing Stew, 175
Quick Lentil and Eggplant Curry, 85
Stir-Fry Toppings, 14

Squash, Winter
Cocoa-Spice Roasted Squash, 69
Cream of Brussels Sprouts Soup with Vegan Cream Sauce, 17
Go-To Winter Medley, 112
Leek and Butternut Squash Soup, 105

Sriracha
Asian-Adzuki Bean Crockpot Chili, 149
Millet, Sunflower Seeds, and Chili-Garlic Sauce, 225

Stevia
High-Fiber Blueberry, Pear, and Spinach Smoothie with Brazil Nuts, 203
Raw Chia Seed Pudding with Cinnamon, 211

Stir-Fry
Carrots Stir-fried with Mung Sprouts and Vegetables, 68
Oyster Mushroom, Asparagus and Tofu Stir Fry, 134
Sesame Bok Choy Shiitake Stir Fry, 7

Simple Shiitake and Broccoli (Mock) Stir-Fry, 139
Stir-Fry Toppings, 14
Tofu and Snow Pea Stir Fry Salad, 101

Strawberries *(see Berries)*

Sundried tomatoes
Greek Garbanzo Bean Salad, 164
Green Beans with Nut Cream Dressing on Minced Tomato Salad, 216
Macadamia Yellow Cheese, 214
Romaine Burritos, 201
Romanesco Broccoli Sauce, 13
Umami Sun-Dried Tomato and Almond Burgers, 202
Veggie Mushroom Burgers, 129

Sweet Potato
Black Bean and Sweet Potato Hash, 152
Curried White and Sweet Potato Pancakes with Fresh Fruit Chutney, 108
Kale and Spring Pea Mash-up, 182
Red Lentil Soup with Sweet Potatoes and Spinach, 176
Rosemary Mushrooms and Kale, 127
Slow Cooker Yellow-Eyed Bean Soup with Sweet Potatoes and Greens, 193
Spicy Red Lentil Vegetable Soup, 177
Split Pea and Yam Soup, 189
Sweet Potato Flatbread, 212

T

Tahini
Creamy House Dressing, 205
Hummus, 165
Kale and Spring Pea Mash-up, 182
Raw Almond Matcha Cakes, 199
Raw Cashew and Tahini Dressing, 206
Rich Mushroom Gravy, 126
Roasted Beet Hummus with Thyme, 82
Root Veggies Paté, 49
Rutabaga "Noodles" with Lemon Balsamic Tahini Sauce, 50
Sesame Bok Choy Shiitake Stir Fry, 7
Summer Arugula Salad with Lemon Tahini Dressing, 6
The Veggie Queen's Raw Kale Salad, 41
Tofu and Snow Pea Stir Fry Salad, 101

Tamari
Brazilian Black Bean Stew (Feijoada), 155
Creamy Ginger-Hemp Dressing, 213

Creamy House Dressing, 205
Grilled Mushroom and Spring Onion Salad with Hummus, 165
Herbed Sesame Crackers, 221
Herby Italian Dressing, 80
Immune Power Soup, 137
Miso Tahini Dressing, 135
Miso Vegetable Soup, 185
Mushroom Un–Meatballs, 138
Pasta with Creamy Cashew Maitake Mushroom Sauce, 132
Protein Powerhouse Trifecta, 150
Rich Mushroom Gravy, 126
Roasted Maitake, 133
Spicy Peanut Citrus Sauce, 217
Taco Nut "Meat", 230
Umami Sun-Dried Tomato and Almond Burgers, 202

Tapioca flour
Coconut-Chickpea Crepes with Smoky Herbed Mushrooms, 122

Tatsoi
Tatsoi with Bok Choy and Mushrooms, 51

Tempeh
Tempeh and Wild Mushroom Stew, 141

Thyme *(see Herbs, Thyme)*

Tofu
Black Bean and Greens Quesadillas with Smoky Chipotle Cream, 151
Creamy Dreamy Broccoli Soup, 11
Garlic Herb Aioli, 99
Garlic, Greens, and Tofu with a Twist, 97
Herbed Tofu Dressing, 80
Lemon Scented Spinach Spread, 103
Oyster Mushroom, Asparagus and Tofu Stir Fry, 134
Potato and Watercress Soup with Sorrel Cream, 55
Thai Bangkok Noodles, 115
Thousand Islands Dressing Sauce, 25
Wild Mushroom Ravioli, 142

Tomatillo
Cilantro Avocado Dressing, 70
Fresh Shelling Beans and Summer Vegetables, 158

Tomato
Asian-Adzuki Bean Crockpot Chili, 149

Baby Leeks a la Nicoise, 104
  Braised Turnip Greens with Tomatoes and
    Thyme, 52
  Chickpea Tomato Soup, 162
  Cream of Brussels Sprouts Soup with Vegan
    Cream Sauce, 17
  Fresh Shelling Beans and Summer Vegetables,
    158
  Garden Bruschetta, 65
  Green Beans with Nut Cream Dressing on
    Minced Tomato Salad, 216
  Leek and Butternut Squash Soup, 105
  Lentil-Leek Soup, 172
  Moroccan Vegetable Tagine, 53
  Quick Lentil and Eggplant Curry, 85
  Raw Cauliflower Tabbouleh, 28
  Shangri-La Soup, 5
  Smoky Sweet Black-Eyed Peas, 159
  Spiced Cauliflower, 72
  Stir-Fry Toppings, 14
  Stuffed Herb Pesto Holiday Appetizers, 67
Tomato paste
  Asian-Adzuki Bean Crockpot Chili, 149
  Herbed Sesame Crackers, 221
  Thousand Islands Dressing Sauce, 25
  Umami Sun-Dried Tomato and Almond
    Burgers, 202
Tomato sauce
  Collard Greens Wrapped Rolls with Spiced
    Quinoa Filling, 33
Tomato, Sundried (see Sundried Tomatoes)
Tortillas
  Black Bean and Greens Quesadillas with
    Smoky Chipotle Cream, 151
Truffles, mushroom
  Truffled Celeriac Soup, 121
Truffles, confection
  Cherry-Chocolate Walnut Truffles, 229
Trumpet Mushrooms (see Mushrooms)
Turmeric (see Spices)
Turnip
  Balsamic Glazed Herb Roasted Roots with
    Kohlrabi, Rutabaga, Turnip, Fennel, Carrots
    and Potatoes, 43
  Moroccan Vegetable Tagine, 53
  Scalloped Turnips Casserole, 54

Stir-Fry Toppings, 14
Turnip greens
  Braised Turnip Greens with Tomatoes and
    Thyme, 52
  Moroccan Vegetable Tagine, 53

V
Vanilla
  Banana Nut Chia Pudding, 209
  Creamy Cashew Almond Custard, 204
  Decadent Chocolate Peanut Butter Truffles, 215
  Hemp Seed Chocolate Mylk, 213
  Overnight Muesli, 210
  Raw Chia Seed Pudding with Cinnamon, 211
Vinegar, balsamic (see Balsamic vinegar)
Vinegar, apple cider
  Black Bean Peanut Butter Brownies, 154
  Herbed Sesame Crackers, 221
  Raw Cashew and Tahini Dressing, 206
Vinegar, red wine
  Baby Leeks a la Nicoise, 104
  Creamy House Dressing, 205
Vinegar, rice wine
  Asian Bean Dip, 190
  Garlic Sesame Broccoli Salad, 99
  Gingered Cucumber Salad, 75
  Herbed Tofu Dressing, 80
  Herby Italian Dressing, 80
  Jill's Mustard Blend, 78
  Pepita Parsnip Paté, 219
  Rice and Veggie Sushi Salad, 186
  Spicy Peanut Citrus Sauce, 217
  Tofu and Snow Pea Stir Fry Salad, 101
Vinegar, ume plum
  Rice and Veggie Sushi Salad, 186

W
Walnuts (see Nuts)
Wasabi
  Rice and Veggie Sushi Salad, 186
Watercress
  Potato and Watercress Soup with Sorrel
    Cream, 55
  Watercress-Sage Pesto, 56
  Sweet Watercress Smoothie, 57
Wheatgrass powder
  Raw Almond Matcha Cakes, 199

White Beans *(see Beans, white)*

White Button Mushrooms *(see Mushrooms)*

Wine
Braised Green Cabbage, 20
Braised Turnip Greens with Tomatoes and
Thyme, 52
Red Lentil Soup with Sweet Potatoes and
Spinach, 176

Y

Yam *(see Sweet Potato)*

Z

Zucchini *(see Squash, Summer)*

RECIPES BY AUTHOR

Asbell, Robin
Pepita Parsnip Paté, 219
Red Lentil Soup with Sweet Potatoes and
Spinach, 176

Bennett, Beverly Lynn
Horseradish and Cannellini Bean Dip, 36
Zesty Broccoli Rabe with Chickpeas and
Pasta, 16
Scalloped Turnips Casserole, 54

Burton, Dreena
Creamy House Dressing, 205
Pumpkin Seed and Chocolate Chip Oatmeal
Breakfast Bars, 218
Umami Sun-Dried Tomato and Almond
Burgers, 202
Wonder Spread, 207

Cerier, Leslie
Falafel Patties, 163

Challis, Tess
Ginger Lime Carrot Soup, 74
Immune Power Soup, 137
Kid's Kale, 39
Pasta with Zesty Lemon White Bean Sauce, 191
Raw Cinnamon Rolls, 230

Chef AJ
Chef AJ's 8 Minute Split Pea Soup, 187
Hail to the Kale Salad, 38
Overnight Muesli, 210

Cook, Shivie
Kale Cabbage Coleslaw with Sunflower Seed
Spicy Thai Dressing, 227

Costiga, Fran
Blueberry Gel, 71

Crawley, Amber Shea
Cherry-Chocolate Walnut Truffles, 229
Roasted Cauliflower and Chickpea Curry, 29

Eccleston, Morgan
Black Bean Collard Wraps, 153
Chickpea Tomato Soup, 162
Garlic Sesame Broccoli Salad, 99
Smoky Collard Greens, 35

Fields, JL
Asian-Adzuki Bean Crockpot Chili, 149
Kale-Apple Slaw with Goji Berry Dressing, 37

Fisher, Cathy
Cabbage Lime Salad with Dijon-Lime
Dressing, 22
Rosemary Mushrooms and Kale, 127
Split Pea and Yam Soup, 189

Forrest, Carrie
Cashew Almond Date Milk, 205
Kale and Spring Pea Mash-up, 182
Sweet Watercress Smoothie, 57

Gillotti, Camina
Summer Seasoning Blend, 87
Fall Seasoning Blend, 88
Winter Seasoning Blend, 88
Spring Seasoning Blend, 88

Greenspan, Sharon
Bok Choy Ginger Dizzle, 7
Hemp Seed Chocolate Mylk, 213
Macadamia Yellow Cheese, 214
Red Almond Cheese, 200

Grossov, Lydia
Braised Green Cabbage, 20
Brazilian Black Bean Stew (Feijoada), 155
Truffled Celeriac Soup, 121

Haney, Nikki
Baked Broccoli Burgers, 10
Creamy Southern Soup Beans, 183

Heino, Katja
Banana Nut Chia Pudding, 209
Grain-Free Just Seeds Crackers, 226
Hazelnut Sesame Bars, 220
Shiitake Mushroom Asparagus Spinach
Soup, 140

Hester, Kathy
Collard Green and Quinoa Taco or Burrito
Filling, 32
Slow Cooker Yellow-Eyed Bean Soup with
Sweet Potatoes and Greens, 193

Jaffe Jones, Ellen
Protein Powerhouse Trifecta, 150
Stir-Fry Toppings, 14
Tuscan Soup with a Twist, 192

Kanner, Ellen
Gutsy Greek Gigantes Beans with Greens,
Oregano and Mint, 79

M'jeddrah, 174
Moroccan Vegetable Tagine, 53
Vegan Red Beans and Rice, 167

Karpovich, Jaime
Chickpea and Strawberry Summer Salad, 161
Leek and Potato Soup, 106
Lemon-Pepper Arugula Pizza with White Bean Basil Sauce, 4

Kingsbury, Judith
Lentil Coconut Spinach Soup, 170
Spicy Red Lentil Vegetable Soup, 177

Long, Linda
Green Beans with Nut Cream Dressing on Minced Tomato Salad, 216
Roasted Stuffed Onions with Carrot-Potato Purée, 113

Lynskey, Jenn
Black Bean and Greens Quesadillas with Smoky Chipotle Cream, 151
Pasta with Creamy Cashew Maitake Mushroom Sauce, 132
Sesame Bok Choy Shiitake Stir Fry, 7
White Bean Garlic Soup, 102

McBride, Kami
Herbed Sesame Crackers, 221
Roasted Beet Hummus with Thyme, 82
Watercress-Sage Pesto, 56

McDougall, Mary
Crunchy Kohlrabi Quinoa Salad, 42
Fennel with Broccoli, Zucchini and Peppers, 12

Moran, Victoria
Chickpea Curry, 160
Shangri-La Soup, 5

Morgan, Christy
Summer Arugula Salad with Lemon Tahini Dressing, 6
Yam Boats with Chickpeas, Bok Choy and Cashew Dill Sauce, 9

Muelrath, Lani
Fat-Free "Forks Over Knives"-Style Onion Mushroom Gravy, 110

Nicholds, Heather
Black Bean Peanut Butter Brownies, 154
Ginger-Pineapple Pudding, 76
Parsley Pistachio Lime Pesto, 81
Rutabaga "Noodles" with Lemon Balsamic Tahini Sauce, 50

Nussinow, Jill
All Purpose Salt-Free Spicy Mix, 89
Allium Broth, 95
Asian Bean Dip, 190
Arugula and Herb Pesto, 3
Baby Leeks a la Nicoise, 104
Balsamic Glazed Herb Roasted Roots with Kohlrabi, Rutabaga, Turnip, Fennel, Carrots and Potatoes, 43
Black Bean and Sweet Potato Hash, 152
Bok Choy, Green Garlic and Greens with Sweet Ginger Sauce, 8
Braised Cabbage with Cumin, 73
Broccoli with Turmeric, Ginger and Garlic, 84
Cabbage and Red Apple Slaw, 21
Cilantro Avocado Dressing, 70
Cocoa Spice Powder, 89
Collard Greens Wrapped Rolls with Spiced Quinoa Filling, 33
Creamy Caesar Salad Dressing, 96
Creamy Ginger-Hemp Dressing, 213
Curried Lentils and Spinach, 169
Curried White and Sweet Potato Pancakes with Fresh Fruit Chutney, 108
Daikon Radish Rawvioli with Creamy Nut Filling, 48
French Green Lentil Salad with Asparagus and Pine Nuts, 173
Fresh Shelling Beans and Summer Vegetables, 158
Garlic, Greens, and Tofu with a Twist, 97
Garlic Herb Aioli, 99
Garlicky Lemon Spinach Salad with Sunflower Seeds, Olives and Sprouted Beans, 100
Gingered Cucumber Salad, 75
Gomasio: Seaweed, Seeds and Salt Sprinkle, 222
Greek Garbanzo Bean Salad, 164
Grilled Mushroom and Spring Onion Salad with Miso Tahini Dressing, 135
Herb and Chile Rub, 90
Herbed Sunflower Seed Dip or Spread with a Fermented "Cheeze" Variation, 228
Herbed Tofu Dressing, 80
Herby Italian Dressing, 80
Hummus, 165
Immune Broth, 136
Jill's Mustard Blend, 78
Lemon Scented Spinach Spread, 103
Lemony Lentil and Potato Chowder, 168
Lentil, Mushroom and Walnut Paté, 123

Lime and Ginger Fruit Salad, 77
Mediterranean Greens, 34
Minted Pea Soup, 179
Miso Vegetable Soup, 185
Mushroom Oat Burgers, 145
Mushroom Un–Meatballs, 138
Mustard Greens, Snow Peas, Green Garlic and
  Kumquats Spring Slaw, 46
Oyster Mushroom, Asparagus and Tofu Stir
  Fry, 134
Pinto Bean Quinoa Burgers, 184
Potato and Watercress Soup with Sorrel
  Cream, 55
Quick Lentil and Eggplant Curry, 85
Rainbow Sprout Salad, 178
Raw Cauliflower Tabbouleh, 28
Rice and Veggie Sushi Salad, 186
Rich Mushroom Gravy, 126
Roasted Maitake, 133
Romanesco Broccoli Sauce, 13
Simple Sauerkraut, 26
Simple Shiitake and Broccoli (Mock) Stir-Fry, 139
Spiced Nuts, 91
Spicy Black Bean Dip, 156
Spicy Peanut Citrus Sauce, 217
Super Spring Salad with Zesty Orange
  Dressing, 77
Tatsoi with Bok Choy and Mushrooms, 51
Tempeh and Wild Mushroom Stew, 141
Thai Bangkok Noodles, 115
Thai-Inspired Broccoli Slaw, 15
Thai Rice, Snow Pea and Mushroom Salad, 180
The Veggie Queen's Husband's Daily Green
  Smoothie, 40
The Veggie Queen's Raw Kale Salad, 41
Tomatillo Black Bean Salsa, 70
Veggie Mushroom Burgers, 129
Wild Mushroom and Farro Stew, 131
Wild Mushroom Ravioli, 142

Patel, Gita
  Carrots Stir-Fried with Mung Sprouts and
    Vegetables, 68
  Spiced Cauliflower, 72

Ranzi, Karen
  No-Bean Hummus, 220
  Root Veggies Paté, 49
  Romaine Burritos, 201
  Stuffed Herb Pesto Holiday Appetizers, 67

Rivera, Rita
  Cashew Almond Date Milk, 205
  Creamy Cashew Almond Custard, 204
  Kale Apple Almond Milk, 199

Robertson, Robin
  Chipotle Cauliflower Mashers, 27
  Roasted Cauliflower with Arugula Pesto, 31

Rodriguez, Elisa
  Easy Salsa Supper, 157
  Go-To Winter Medley, 112
  Kale Apply Curry, 86
  Nourishing Stew, 175

Schinner, Miyoko
  Mango, Daikon, and Avocado Spring Rolls, 49
  Mushroom Thyme Sauce, 83
  Trumpet Mushroom and Avocado Ceviche, 144

Scott-Hamilton, Carolyn
  Decadent Chocolate Peanut Butter Truffles, 215
  Garden Bruschetta, 65
  Sweet Potato Flatbread, 212
  Taco Nut "Meat", 230
  Tofu and Snow Pea Stir Fry Salad, 101

Sutton, Mark
  "Maizing" Brassica Pizza, 223
  Really Reubenesque Revisited Pizza, 23

Theodore, Laura
  Leek and Butternut Squash Soup, 105
  Quick-Stuffed Crimini Mushrooms, 125

Valpone, Amie
  Cinnamon Roasted Radishes, 47
  Roasted Turmeric Brussels Sprouts with Hemp
    Seeds on Arugula, 19

Williams, Joanne Mumola
  High-Fiber Blueberry, Pear, and Spinach
    Smoothie with Brazil Nuts, 203
  Kidney Bean Salad with Chili-Lime Dressing, 166
  Lentil-Leek Soup, 172
  Raw Chia Seed Pudding with Cinnamon, 211

Wyrick, Jason
  Mustard Greens and Gumbo, 44
  Smoked Trumpet Mushroom Potato Soup, 143

Wysocarski, Erin
  Coconut-Chickpea Crepes with Smoky Herbed
    Mushrooms, 122
  Raw Almond Matcha Cakes, 199
  Raw Cashew and Tahini Dressing, 206

Jill Nussinow, MS, RD

PO Box 6042, Santa Rosa, CA 95406-0042
1-800-919-1VEG (834) theveggiequeen.com

Jill's Other Books

The Veggie Queen™: Vegetables Get the Royal Treatment

*The New Fast Food:™ The Veggie Queen Pressure Cooks
Whole Food Meals in Less than 30 Minutes*

Jill's DVDs:

Pressure Cooking: A Fresh Look, Delicious Dishes in Minutes

Creative Low-Fat Vegan Cuisine

You can find The Veggie Queen videos online at:
www.youtube.com/TheVQ

To sign up for my email newsletter or to order more books,
please go to my website at: **www.theveggiequeen.com**

Discounts are available for orders of 10 or more copies.

I am available to speak to your group, to teach a cooking class, do cooking
demonstrations or help plan weekend retreats for your group. Just ask.

CPSIA information can be obtained at www.ICGtesting.com
Printed in the USA
BVOW09s1656310714

360617BV00003B/8/P